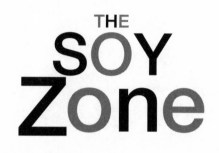

Other books by Barry Sears

The Zone

Mastering the Zone

Zone-Perfect Meals in Minutes

Zone Food Blocks

The Anti-Aging Zone

A Week in the Zone

THE
SOY
Zone

Barry Sears, Ph.D.

ReganBooks
An Imprint of HarperCollins*Publishers*

This book is not intended to replace medical advice or be a substitute for a physician. If you are sick or suspect you are sick, you should see a physician. If you are taking a prescription medication, you should never change your diet (for better or worse) without consulting your physician, because any dietary change will affect the metabolism of that prescription drug.

Prevention will always be the best medicine. However, prevention can only be undertaken by the individual, and that includes eating correctly. This is the foundation of a healthy lifestyle. You have to eat, so you may as well eat wisely.

Although this book is about food, the author and the publisher expressly disclaim responsibility for any adverse effects arising from following the advice given in this book without appropriate medical supervision.

THE SOY ZONE. Copyright © 2000 by Barry Sears, Ph.D. All rights reserved. Printed in the United States of America. No part of this book may be used or reproduced in any manner whatsoever without written permission except in the case of brief quotations embodied in critical articles and reviews. For information address HarperCollins Publishers Inc., 10 East 53rd Street, New York, NY 10022.

HarperCollins books may be purchased for educational, business, or sales promotional use. For information please write: Special Markets Department, HarperCollins Publishers Inc., 10 East 53rd Street, New York, NY 10022.

FIRST EDITION

Designed by Nancy Singer Olaguera

Printed on acid-free paper

Library of Congress Cataloging-in-Publication Data has been applied for.

ISBN 0-06-039310-6

00 01 02 03 04 ❖/RRD 10 9 8 7 6 5 4 3 2 1

contents

Appendixes

acknowledgments

The success of the Zone books that I have written during the past five years is primarily due to my team, who are not only my co-workers, but also my closest friends. These include my wife, Lynn Sears, who does much of the editing of my books, and my brother, Doug Sears, who has a very clear insight and understanding of how to translate cutting-edge science into easily understood terms for the general public. In addition, I wish to especially thank Deborah Kotz for her excellent advice and input in helping develop this book and Jill Sullivan for her insightful comments.

Special thanks go to Roberto Mighty, who orchestrated the various soy recipes from a variety of talented Soy Zone chefs. It is the expertise of these chefs that makes it easy to integrate the Soy Zone into your daily lifestyle. These Zone chefs include Rachel Albert-Matesz, who is a cookbook author and has written more than 150 articles that have appeared in such magazines as *Vegetarian Times, Vegetarian Gourmet, Veggie Life,* and *Vegetarian Journal.* Also among these Soy Zone chefs are Janet Candela, a longtime vegetarian chef, and Shoshana Levinson, who holds a master's degree in human nutrition and biology and is a certified nutrition specialist in Connecticut. Her nutrition counseling services are focused on weight management and the treatment of chronic conditions such as diabetes, heart disease, allergies, and digestive disorders. Finally, there is my long-term colleague Dr. René Espy, who uses many soy-based Zone meals for her patients.

At the same time, I also have a team at ReganBooks that consistently does an outstanding job of fine-tuning my books for the general public. For this particular book, I want to give special thanks to Vanessa Stich, Cassie Jones, Renée Iwaszkiewicz, and Doug Corcoran for their excellent editing.

Of course, my greatest thanks always go to Judith Regan, who had the courage and foresight to support the Zone, and in the process helped improve the lives of millions of people.

introduction

Do you want to live a longer and healthier life? I know I do. Unfortunately, I am also genetically programmed for an early heart attack. For the past two generations most of the males in my family have died of heart attacks by their mid-fifties. I have inherited these same poor genes.

I can't change my genes, but perhaps I *can* change my genetic destiny by altering the expression of certain genes through the foods I eat. This may sound like scientific fantasy, but it turns out that food is the most potent medicine of all. This is because food can indirectly turn certain genes on and off by altering levels of hormones. I have spent nearly 20 years researching how the foods we eat affect our hormones and how these hormones alter our genetic fate. I hope the scientific odyssey I have embarked upon to prolong the length and quality of my own life can help you do the same.

The basis of the Zone Diet comes from my background in the development of intravenous delivery systems for cancer drugs. I learned that if too little of the drug is administered, the patient dies of cancer. If the patient gets too much, he will die from the drug's toxicity. The goal of the cancer treatment is to maintain that drug within a therapeutic zone: not too high, not too low. I realized that the same philosophy was relevant to maintaining food-generated hormones in similar zones, and our success in reaching that goal depends on the balance of protein, carbohydrate, and fat we eat at every meal.

The Soy Zone represents the next chapter of my ongoing scientific journey, which I have chronicled in all the Zone books I have written in the last five years. This book will explain how following the Zone Diet using primarily soy protein will move you closer to that elusive goal of a longer and better life. It will also bring you vast benefits right now: You'll have more energy and a sharper mental focus to tackle your daily challenges. You'll also shed excess body fat, and keep it off for life. Without a doubt, the Soy Zone Diet is the most powerful version of my Zone technology that I have developed. What's more, the Soy Zone is ideally suited for vegetarians (even vegans) who want to enter the Zone.

The humble soybean is now being hailed as the next magic bullet that will help save us. In many ways that statement is true, because as we replace more of the animal protein in our diet with soy protein, better health is assured. However, if your goal is living longer and better, that can only be achieved by ensuring that your overall diet is hormonally correct, and that means keeping your hormones within a defined zone: not too high, not too low. In other words, you need to combine all the health benefits of soy with a hormonal balancing system like the Zone. When you do, you enter the Soy Zone—which I believe is the healthiest diet in the world.

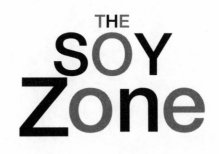

THE
SOY
Zone

The Health Benefits of Soy

"Why do I need to get into the Zone?" That's a question I've been asked a thousand times, and it's a question that runs through my mind every day as I conduct research and lecture across the country about the benefits of the Zone. I usually answer this question with a question of my own:

Do you want to live a longer and healthier life?

You've probably heard that "you are what you eat" and that a nutritious diet is the key to good health. In this day and age, we are faced with a plethora of conflicting dietary advice and an overwhelming number of food choices. If you avoid all fat, do you still need to worry about calories? Is a high-carbohydrate diet the way to go? Or are high-protein diets the best choice?

Let's face it: You're probably more confused than ever about what to eat. In fact, most Americans don't know which way to turn and, as a result of heeding bad nutritional advice, we're in the midst of a growing obesity epidemic—with more than 50 percent of us overweight.

Let's cut through all the nutribabble and focus on one thing: If you balance the foods you eat, you achieve balance in your body, which will lead to a longer and healthier life. The Zone Diet contains the balance of carbohydrates, protein, and fat that will take you 90 percent of the way there. If you replace some of the low-fat animal protein (meat, chicken, fish, dairy, egg whites) from the Zone Diet with soy protein, you'll get the rest of the way there.

I believe the Soy Zone is the healthiest diet in the world—a diet that creates balance in your body's hormonal systems and keeps your body running at peak efficiency. You'll feel healthier and will have a lower risk of developing such life-threatening diseases as heart disease, cancer, and diabetes. At the same time, you'll experience more energy and a mental sharpness that will carry you through the day. If you're overweight, the Soy Zone is a perfect way to shed excess fat and keep it off for life.

It's time to enter the Soy Zone.

The Soy Zone Diet is the most advanced form of the Zone. What is the Zone? It is the *balance* of hormonal systems that occurs every time you eat. You can enter the Zone by balancing the foods you eat through a diet program that I introduced in my 1995 book, *The Zone,* and refined in my 1997 book, *Mastering the Zone.* The Zone is a protein-adequate diet in which you consume about 40 percent of your calories from carbohydrates, about 30 percent from protein, and 30 percent from fat. As you can see, this diet is neither high-protein nor high-carbohydrate. It's a diet that restores the proper balance of protein, carbohydrate, and fat, a balance your body needs to work effectively.

The Zone is not some mythical place or catchy marketing slogan. The basic premise of the Zone is that eating the proper balance of foods will keep certain hormones within a therapeutic zone. What's amazing is that you can precisely control how your body functions through the foods you eat. You can help extend your lifespan and prevent chronic disease.

So where does soy fit in? Soy is a natural form of plant protein that fits perfectly into the Zone Diet. In fact, it actually enhances the effects of the Zone, making it easier to achieve the hormonal balance that your body needs. If you're familiar with the rules of the Zone, you'll find it easy to adopt the Soy Zone. All you need to do is replace some of the low-fat animal protein you normally eat with soy protein products. If you've never tried the Zone, simply follow the step-by-step rules outlined in the next chapter. You'll see that it won't take much effort to get into the Zone. And once you're there, you'll want to stay there.

Over the past few years, soy food products have become extremely popular in this country. Newspaper headlines tout study after study showing the health benefits of soy. Sure, you'd like to try some soy foods—if you haven't already. But maybe you've stared quizzically at the package of tofu or soy hamburger crumbles on the supermarket shelf, wondering how to incorporate these foods into your favorite dishes.

It's for you that I wrote this book. You'll find this book extremely useful if you fall into one of these three categories:

- You want to add more soy to your diet because you've heard it's healthy, but you consider this dietary change too difficult, restrictive, or time-consuming. I will show you how to make a wide variety of gourmet soy-based meals that are simple to prepare, yet elegant to both the eye and the palate. More importantly, each Soy Zone meal is guaranteed to put you into the Zone for a four- to six-hour period.

- You already follow the Zone Diet, but you want a greater number of soy-based meals to give you some more variety and to give you the maximum amount of control over your hormones.

- You are a vegetarian and have not experienced the promised benefits of a vegetarian lifestyle. Maybe you're getting fatter, losing strength, or are constantly fatigued. You don't need to give up your vegetarian lifestyle or continue to live feeling rundown. You simply need to make some simple adjustments, such as adding soy protein to your diet and reducing the amount of grains you eat. These changes will shoot you straight into the Zone.

The Problem with the Traditional Vegetarian Diet

Traditional vegetarian diets rely heavily on grains and starches, with relatively little protein. These diets are hormonally unbalanced because they contain huge amounts of carbohydrates and little else. Eating a diet based almost solely on carbohydrates causes insulin levels to soar, which causes blood sugar levels to drop quickly. As a result, many vegetarians find themselves feeling sluggish and always searching for more food (primarily more carbohydrates to temporarily restore blood sugar levels). They may also find themselves gaining weight. The insidious long-term consequence of a grain-based vegetarian diet is the constant elevation of insulin levels. Unfortunately, this diet is commonly recommended to people with heart disease, diabetes, and cancer—all diseases that are associated with elevated insulin levels.

WHAT YOU CAN EXPECT AFTER TWO WEEKS IN THE SOY ZONE

Once you begin following the Soy Zone Diet, you'll experience some immediate benefits—within the first two weeks. Here's what you can look forward to. You will:

1. **Think better.** By keeping your blood sugar levels stable throughout the day, you'll find you have a better ability to concentrate and won't have that mental haziness that can occur around two to three hours after eating a high-carbohydrate meal.

2. **Have increased energy.** Eating more (but not excessive) protein will increase your levels of the hormone glucagon, which enables your body to maintain constant blood sugar levels for mental energy. You will feel more refreshed in the morning and more energized throughout the day. Afternoon mental slumps will be a thing of the past.

3. **Look better as your clothes begin to fit better.** Of course, you can't expect to lose 10 pounds during the first week, but you probably will lose about 1 to 2 pounds of fat and about 2 to 3 pounds of

retained water—up to 5 pounds total. The retained water is due to excess insulin levels, which are lowered as you switch to fewer carbohydrates and more protein.

4. **Feel a greater sense of well-being.** You'll feel less cranky and moody between meals because you won't experience those sugar lows that make you tired, hungry, and irritable. Overall, you'll feel like your life is on an even keel—a sign that your hormones are, too.

5. **Experience fewer carbohydrate cravings.** On the Soy Zone Diet, you'll be eating fewer calories than you're used to but won't feel as hungry. Resetting your hormonal balance will regulate your blood sugar levels, so you won't be craving carbohydrates for short-term energy.

6. **Fine-tune your insulin levels.** Several recent research findings suggest that following the Zone Diet can result in an almost immediate reduction of elevated insulin levels, which is the underlying cause of diabetes and heart disease. A 1998 study from Australia found that diabetics who followed the Zone Diet for three days experienced a 36 percent decrease in their insulin levels. In the same study, overweight but nondiabetic individuals had a 40 percent decrease in their elevated insulin levels. A more recent study from Harvard Medical School found that the insulin-controlling benefits kick in after just one meal in the Zone.

You'll think better throughout the day because you will maintain constant blood sugar levels, which the brain needs to sustain mental acuity (think of how tired and fuzzy you feel two to three hours after eating a big bowl of pasta). For the same biochemical reason, you won't be hungry, since the brain is getting all the fuel it needs. You'll perform better because you'll be able to gain access to your stored body fat and burn it off as a virtually unlimited source of energy. You'll look better because you will lose excess body fat while maintaining your muscle mass. Although you won't see a huge change immediately on your bathroom scale, your clothes will fit much better as your body composition changes to what it was at a younger age. You'll get all of these benefits plus the vastly increased likelihood of living longer. It's not a bad trade-off for making some very simple changes in your diet.

THE SOY SOLUTION

In the 1970s, tofu was the new hot fad food appearing in trendy restaurants across the United States. We mixed the soy product into stir-fry vegetables and mashed it into egg salads, but we quickly realized it was too bland to eat on its own. Tofu fell from favor for a time, but fortunately recent advances in the food industry have ushered in a resurgence of soy.

There are now literally hundreds of products on supermarket shelves that contain soy protein—from veggie burgers to nondairy cheese to meatless ground beef. You can find soybeans mixed into name-brand frozen vegetables or eat them dried as soy nuts. You can cook with tempeh and soy flour in addition to tofu. Chapter 3 contains a full list of the types of soy products available, how you can use them, and where you can find them.

The rise in soy products came about from the public's demand for nutritious, low-fat foods that are high in protein and—above all—don't force them to sacrifice taste. Soybeans are the only vegetables that contain more protein than carbohydrate, making them the perfect way to get an adequate amount of protein through a vegetarian meal. Soybeans are virtually a complete protein, providing much of the essential amino acids, those components of protein that you need to get through your diet in order to stay healthy. However, your body is better able to absorb the protein from soybean products that are highly processed (like protein powders, tofu, and tempeh) than from natural soybeans. In fact, the amino acids in processed soy products are nearly equivalent in quality to the amino acids found in meat, milk, and egg protein. For this reason, I don't think you can get the full benefits of the Soy Zone without including some processed soy products in your diet, which are included in my list of soy foods in Chapter 3.

Besides being rich in protein, soy has unique properties that help your body maintain steady insulin levels even better than other protein-rich foods, such as meat or chicken. Although I'll get into more detail about how this happens later in the book, here's the reason why in a nutshell: Soy is rich in an amino acid that causes your body to release the hormone glucagon—the anti-insulin hormone—that mobilizes stored carbohydrates from the liver to keep your body supplied with energy, thereby eliminating hunger. It also contains much less of "bad-guy" amino acids, which trigger the release of insulin.

Soy has another added plus: It contains isoflavones, which are disease-fighting substances (called phytochemicals) found only in plants. These isoflavones mimic the female hormone estrogen. Research suggests that these isoflavones may ward off a variety of diseases from heart disease to cancer to osteoporosis and to alleviate hot flashes and other menopausal symptoms.

Recognizing the wide body of research showing the health benefits of soy, the U.S. government recommends that everyone eat 25 grams of soy a day (about half the amount of soy recommended on the Soy Zone, but it's a start). What's more, the Food and Drug Administration last year decided to allow some of the health benefits of soy to be touted on food labels. Products that contain a substantial amount of soy protein can claim that they may reduce the risk of heart disease. Without a doubt, soy packs a powerful nutritional punch that will boost the health benefits from the Zone to new heights. Consider this summary of the latest research:

HEALTH BENEFITS OF SOY

In recent years, researchers have become aware of the vast health benefits of eating soy foods, mostly by studying populations throughout the world who eat a lot of soy. Although these studies don't necessarily prove that soybeans are the magic elixir of life, they definitely suggest that soy confers certain health benefits on people who consume a lot of it. Here are some of specific benefits that have been attributed to soy:

- **Reduces the risk of heart disease.** It's well known that in countries where soy products are eaten regularly, rates of heart disease are low. For the past 30 years, researchers have shown that consuming soy products causes a decrease in both total cholesterol and LDL ("bad") cholesterol levels. An analysis of 38 clinical studies published in *The New England Journal of Medicine* in 1995 found that consuming an average of 50 grams of soy per day lowered cholesterol levels by 9 percent. This level of cholesterol reduction should lead to a 20 percent reduction in heart disease risk.

- **Protects Against Breast Cancer.** Breast cancer occurs much less commonly in Asian countries where diets are rich in soy. For instance, Japanese women have only one-quarter the rate of breast cancer of American women.

- **Reduces Risk of Prostate Cancer.** Rates of prostate cancer mortality are far lower in Japanese males (who consume large amounts of soy) than they are in American males.

- **Diminishes Menopausal Symptoms.** Recent research has shown that soy foods may be able to ease most menopausal symptoms, such as night sweats and hot flashes. In one study, night sweats and hot flashes were reduced by 40 percent in women who ate soy foods. Soy contains compounds (isoflavones) that can act as estrogens to help compensate for decreased natural estrogen production during menopause.

- **Helps Prevent Osteoporosis.** It has been shown that a diet rich in soy protein decreases the rate of bone loss, and in one study soy protein consumption actually increased bone density. Beyond isoflavones, some soy products pack a wallop of bone-building calcium. One cup of tofu contains about 20 percent (204 mg) of the U.S. Recommended Daily Allowance (RDA), and one cup of tempeh contains 15 percent (154 mg) of the RDA.

Note: Heart disease, cancer, menopause, and osteoporosis are all complex disease conditions that are intimately connected with the overall diet. Soy protein does, indeed, have some very profound health benefits, but only if used as the cornerstone of a balanced diet like the Zone.

THE QUEST FOR A LONGER LIFE

Rather than assuming what type of diet is best for longevity, I believe it makes more sense to examine different cultures with very different dietary habits and then study the direct relationship of their diets to longevity. Therefore, let's start with a simple question: What do the longest-living people in the world actually eat?

You might think the longest-living people are found eating yogurt in the upper valleys of Tibet or the mountains of southern Russia. These reports of incredible longevity were later found to be false based on the natural propensity of the elderly to exaggerate their age, coupled with a lack of reliable birth records.

Longevity can be defined as the decreased likelihood of dying, which is reflected in a population's death rate. The lower the death rate or mortality, the greater the longevity. By focusing on adults (between the ages of 35 and 74), many of the complicating factors of infant and childhood mortality are eliminated. Once these factors are eliminated, we can assume that whichever population has the lowest death rate is also the one that has the optimal diet to follow for longevity.

So let's examine four very distinct regions of the world with four very distinct diets:

1. Rural Chinese, who eat primarily a grain-based vegetarian diet with limited amounts of protein (but much of it comes from soy),

2. Americans, who eat too much of everything,

3. French, who eat the most elegant food in Europe, and

4. Japanese, who eat a diet rich in soy protein and fish.

The American Heart Association in its 1997 American Heart Association's *Statistical Supplement* compiled the mortality rates for both men and women in these very distinct regions with equally distinctive dietary habits, as shown in the table below.

Mortality Rates (per 100,000) of Adults (Ages 35 to 74)		
Country	**Male Death Rate**	**Female Death Rate**
Rural China	1,433	914
United States	1,209	688
France	1,065	438
Japan	814	380

The rural Chinese, who eat a traditional grain-based vegetarian diet (even though it does contain some soy protein), actually had the highest death rate. One reason might be their lack of adequate protein. An efficient immune system requires adequate levels of protein to maintain its constant battle against infectious agents.

Americans do a little better in terms of decreased mortality compared to the rural Chinese. The increased levels of protein in the American diet compared to the rural Chinese diet may be an important reason for the decrease in the overall adult mortality rate. However, we still consume too many calories, and many of these calories consist of high-density carbohydrates, such as rice, pasta, and breads. Of course, Americans spend a far greater amount of money on health care resources, especially those heroic measures that prolong life. So perhaps our improved mortality is simply a consequence of our extraordinary health care spending.

What about the French? No one has ever accused the French of not eating well, and if you look at the mortality data, they also seem to live longer and probably better than either the rural Chinese or Americans.

Compared to the American diet, the French diet consists of adequate (but not excessive) amounts of protein, and contains far more low-density carbohydrates (fruits and vegetables). Furthermore, the French lack a fear of fat. The end result? The French have the lowest rates of heart disease in Europe, look good in designer clothing, and spend much less of their gross national product on health care compared to Americans. So simply spending more money on health care is not the answer to increased longevity.

Finally, it might appear that the Japanese are the ultimate winners in the longevity race. Unlike the rural Chinese diet, the Japanese diet is more protein-rich (they eat three times as much soy protein and more fish) and contains higher amounts of low-density carbohydrates, such as vegetables, coupled with a corresponding decrease in total rice consumption. In fact, the dramatic increase in Japanese longevity after World War II has been attributed to the combination of increased protein consumption and the reduced rice content of their diet. And like the French, the Japanese spend a much smaller amount of their gross national product on health care compared to Americans.

THE LONGEST-LIVING PEOPLE IN THE WORLD

There is, however, a group of people that lives even longer than the Japanese. Therefore, whatever they eat should be the template for determining the composition of the ideal diet to increase longevity. These people live on the island of Okinawa, which is part of Japan, but separated by 400 miles of ocean. The Okinawans have an adult age-adjusted death rate that is approximately one-half of the overall mainland Japanese population, and they have a larger percentage of the elderly reaching age 100 than any other region in the world.

So what distinguishes the Okinawan diet from the typical mainland Japanese diet? First, they eat more soy protein (see chart on page 12).

As you can quickly see, the Okinawans eat much more soy protein than Americans or mainland Japanese. This can partly explain their incredible longevity because populations that consume greater amounts of soy protein have significantly decreased rates of heart disease, cancer

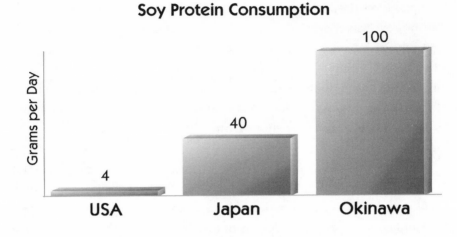

Soy Protein Consumption

(both breast and prostate), and decreased osteoporosis. I will explain later in this book the actual biochemical mechanisms that make soy protein such a potentially powerful therapeutic agent. Obviously, a decrease of any one of these disease conditions would have a positive and very significant impact on longevity.

What is not initially obvious is that the Okinawans consume a lot of total protein, even though much of it is soy protein. Compared to mainland Japanese, they eat twice as much fish, which gives them a hefty dose of heart-healthy long-chain Omega-3 fatty acids. The Okinawans also eat two to three times more vegetables than the mainland Japanese.

However, I feel that the most important factor for Okinawan longevity is that they consume 20 to 40 percent fewer calories than the Japanese. How is it possible to eat more soy protein, fish, and vegetables but consume fewer calories? The answer is simple: they eat fewer *high-density* carbohydrates, such as rice, than the Japanese do.

Reducing calories while maintaining adequate levels of protein, essential fats, plus vitamins and minerals is referred to as *calorie restriction.* Calorie restriction is not malnutrition, since your body isn't deprived of any essential nutrients. It is, though, the only proven way to increase longevity. There is no disagreement (a rarity in scientific circles) in the world of longevity research that calorie restriction works in every animal species tested. And the longevity of the Okinawans appears to indicate that it works in humans. Although the Okinawans eat fewer calories, they have the highest consumption of soy protein of any population in the world. Compared to their fairly healthy Japanese counterparts, the Okinawans have nearly five times the percentage of people living over 100, and have a 30 to 40 percent lower death rate in every age range from heart disease, strokes, and cancer.

This is why the Soy Zone Diet is based on the Okinawan diet, although I adapted it to meet the tastes and needs of most Americans. Like the Okinawan diet, the foundation of the Soy Zone Diet is a combination of consuming more soy protein and more vegetables and increasing the intake of long-chain Omega-3 fatty acids. It hinges on dramatically reducing the amount of grains, starches, and refined carbohydrates that you currently eat. Although cutting calories may sound like a dreadful prospect, you'll actually find that by following the Soy Zone Diet, you'll eat fewer calories without feeling hungry or deprived. With better hormonal control, you'll see excess body fat melt away as your energy levels soar. You'll also experience a dramatic improvement in your health.

The Soy Zone Diet is a lifelong eating strategy designed to prevent those chronic diseases (heart disease, diabetes, cancer, etc.) that are associated with excess insulin production. The Soy Zone involves much more than eating more soy protein. In the next chapter, I'll explain the basic rules of the Soy Zone, and in subsequent chapters, I'll tell you how to stock your kitchen and how to plan your meals. This book also contains breakfast, lunch, dinner, and snack recipes to help you plan a month of Soy Zone meals. If you follow the guidelines in this book, then that elusive goal of living a longer, leaner, and healthier life will become a reality.

What I don't want, though, is for you to take my word for it and follow this plan blindly. I want you to understand why the Soy Zone provides such powerful benefits. The latter half of the book is devoted to increasing your understanding of why you're making the effort to change the way you eat and live. Once you understand how the Soy

Zone works, you'll realize that this book is not some new fad diet, but a powerful therapeutic drug.

Hippocrates once said, "Let food be your medicine, and let medicine be your food." I'm writing you a prescription for the Soy Zone because I know it's the most effective drug for gaining a longer and healthier life.

Enter the Soy Zone

When it comes to the Soy Zone, I practice what I preach. I'm not a strict vegetarian, so I vary my diet between eating Zone meals and Soy Zone meals. Still, I always try to incorporate at least two Soy Zone meals a day in order to get enough soy protein to get its health benefits.

My typical Soy Zone meals might include a soy protein smoothie for breakfast (a blended mixture of soy protein powder, berries, and ground nuts). For lunch, I might have two soy hamburgers, some hummus (mashed chickpeas and olive oil), some steamed vegetables, and a piece of fruit for dessert. For dinner, I could make some chili by sautéing soy hamburger crumbles in olive oil and then adding some salsa and black beans and a side of sautéed vegetables with mixed berries for dessert.

Hard to believe that such a nutritious diet could be so easy to prepare? Truth is, once you change the way you think about food, you'll find that preparing a Soy Zone meal is a snap. First, though, you need to understand why your body needs the balance found in the Zone, and the rules you need to follow that will take you into the Zone.

GETTING YOUR BODY BALANCED GIVES YOU CONTROL

Being in the Zone puts you in the driver's seat and literally takes away your enslavement to food. The Zone is not some mystical place, but a state of hormonal balance that can only be achieved by the food you

15

eat. You may see yourself as a victim to the foods you crave. If you're feeling down and draggy, you down some cookies or potato chips to give yourself some energy and help you feel a little better. This measure, though, only works temporarily, and you're soon left feeling even more tired after the short-term surge in energy wears off. You may feel like a strung-out addict looking for another fix. In a sense you are, but now you're looking for a fix of carbohydrates. This off-balance, out-of-control feeling is simply a consequence of your hormones being out of balance. If you want to break this habit, you have to get into the Zone.

The high-carbohydrate diet that most Americans live on is a hormonally unbalanced one. From a physiological standpoint, a diet filled with bread, pasta, rice, and cereals will send your insulin levels soaring and keep them elevated throughout the day. This is because any carbohydrate must be broken down into the simplest form of sugar, known as *glucose,* to be absorbed. As these carbohydrates enter the bloodstream, you may feel euphoric, but you only feel this way temporarily, until your insulin levels shoot up. Insulin's job is to drive nutrients like blood sugar to the cells, and once it does its work, you're left feeling just as hungry and tired as before. As a form of self-medication, you consume more carbohydrates, and start the cycle over again. The end result is that you gain weight and put yourself at greater risk for heart disease, diabetes, and cancer because of the constant elevation of insulin levels.

For years, I've been frustrated by the all-out war we've been waging against dietary fat as opposed to excess insulin. Although you do need some insulin to deliver nutrients to your cells, excess insulin can be extraordinarily dangerous to your health. Not only will it cause your body to store any excess calories as fat, but it also disrupts a wide variety of other hormonal systems and eventually leads to the development of chronic disease. The bottom line is, the more excess insulin you make, the fatter you become and the more likely you are to die at an earlier age.

Being in the Zone means that you have stabilized your insulin and blood sugar levels, so that they're not flip-flopping from high to low and low to high. If you follow the rules of the *Soy Zone Diet,* you will be able to control your insulin, so that you won't feel hungry between meals, and you won't crave the food that your body doesn't need.

How do you get to the Zone? Ironically, reaching it is based on two words your grandmother emphasized: *balance* and *moderation*. Eating a balanced meal containing a moderate number of calories is the key to getting into the Zone. Here are the basic rules of the Soy Zone Diet.

RULE #1: ALWAYS KEEP A BALANCE OF PROTEIN AND CARBOHYDRATE EVERY TIME YOU EAT

At every meal or snack, you need to eat a mixture of protein and carbohydrates to maintain steady insulin levels. Although fat has no effect on insulin, you need to have a little mixed into every meal and snack because it helps slow down the entry rate of carbohydrates into the bloodstream, which will indirectly lower the insulin response of a meal. Fat also sends a signal to the brain that says, "Stop eating, you're full." Finally, fat makes food taste better (ask the French). So, every time you eat, you need to have the *right* mix of protein and carbohydrate and a dash of fat. The result will be a steady zone of insulin for the next four to six hours.

How do you get the right mixture of protein and carbohydrates? Simply divide your plate into three parts. If you're eating a Soy Zone breakfast, lunch, or dinner, use a standard dinner plate. If you're eating a Soy Zone snack, use a dessert plate (see figure below).

Divide Your Plate Into 3 Sections

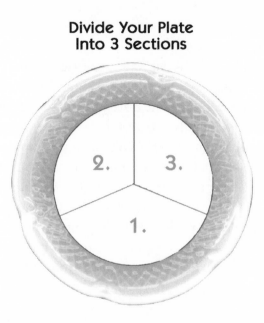

To prepare a Soy Zone meal, fill one-third of your plate primarily with soy protein: this could be tofu or a soybean meat substitute product. Lacto-ovo vegetarians (those who eat eggs and dairy products) can also add small amounts of low-fat egg and dairy products to this low-fat soy protein section of the plate. Non-vegetarians can add small amounts of low-fat protein sources, like fish and chicken, to the low-fat soy protein section as shown in the figure below. The amount of protein you have on your plate should equal about the size and thickness of your palm.

Start with Low-Fat Protein . . .

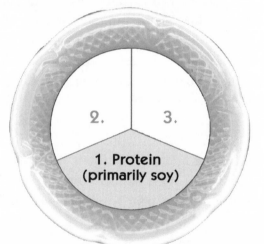

2.

3.

1. Protein
(primarily soy)

Fill the other two-thirds of your plate (see figure) with carbohydrates—primarily with vegetables, and to a lesser extent fruit. If you really want pasta, rice, a potato or some other starch, fill just one-third of the plate with these types of carbohydrates and leave the other third of your plate empty (just make sure that the volume of the starch is the same volume as the protein on your plate). I recommend doing this only occasionally, because you will get far more nutrients (not to mention better insulin control) from a plate filled with vegetables and fruit than from one filled with grains or starches. On a volume basis, grains contain far fewer nutrients and far greater amounts of carbohydrates than vegetables and fruits. This is why they are used as condiments on the Soy Zone Diet.

**Fill other sections with vegetables
and some fruits**

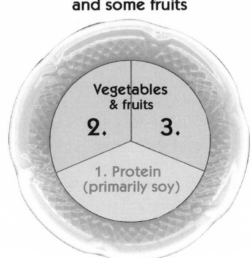

The last item is fat: Just add a small amount of monounsaturated fat—the heart-healthy kind that's found in olive oil, selected nuts, and avocados. Sauté your vegetables in two teaspoons of olive oil, sprinkle on a handful of slivered almonds, or cut in an eighth of an avocado. As you can see, the amount of fat used in the Soy Zone is not that much. Of course, you should avoid saturated fats and trans fats (partially hydrogenated oils) because they can increase cholesterol levels and contribute to an increased risk of heart disease.

Notice that at no time during the preparation of a Soy Zone meal have you counted calories or grams or made complex calculations. All you used was your eye and the palm of your hand.

RULE #2: GO FOR LOW-DENSITY CARBOHYDRATES, RATHER THAN HIGH-DENSITY CARBOHYDRATES

Unless you're familiar with my other Zone books, you probably have no idea what this rule means. Basically, I'm telling you to stock up on vegetables and fruit rather than pasta, bagels, and rice. You may not realize that any food that's not a protein or fat is a carbohydrate. Yes, fruits and vegetables are carbohydrates, along with cakes, cookies, cereals, pasta, and starches like potatoes.

Why, then, can't you eat whatever carbohydrate you want as long as you mix it with protein? The answer is that you possibly could, as long as you maintain the balance of protein to carbohydrate. You see, the amount of carbohydrate in a quarter of a candy bar or a quarter cup of cooked pasta is the same as in two cups of stir-fried vegetables or a cup of fresh berries. However, their effects on insulin are very different. High-density carbohydrates (like refined sugars or starches) have much less fiber than low-density carbohydrates (fruits and vegetables). Fiber slows down the entry rate of any carbohydrate into the bloodstream, and that lowers insulin secretion. Second, low-density carbohydrates are the true powerhouses of vitamins and minerals. Finally, low-density carbohydrates take up a lot of room on your plate, so you never feel deprived at any meal.

Vegetables should be your primary source of carbohydrates on the Soy Zone Diet, supplemented with lesser amounts of fruits, which are higher in carbohydrate density. Following the Soy Zone, you'll have a difficult time overconsuming carbohydrates. On the other hand, we all know how easy it is to eat an extra slice of bread or a second helping of pasta. Unfortunately, the higher amounts of carbohydrates in these little extras will elevate your insulin and shoot you right out of the Zone. By following the Soy Zone Diet, you are using a very elegant control mechanism developed over millions of years of evolution to help keep your insulin levels balanced.

RULE #3: EAT MODERATE PORTIONS

As I describe in great detail in *The Anti-Aging Zone*, the fewer calories you eat, the slower you age and the greater your longevity. This is why the size of a typical Soy Zone meal is approximately 300 calories for a female and 400 calories for a male. Following the Soy Zone Diet, every day you will consume adequate amounts of soy protein, extraordinary levels of vitamins and minerals from low-density carbohydrates (vegetables and fruits), and about 40 to 60 grams of heart-healthy monounsaturated fat, the same amount of fat usually consumed on most vegetarian diets. Yet you'll only be eating around 1,200 calories a day if you're a woman, and 1,500 calories a day if you're a man.

What's amazing, though, is that you can consume fewer calories on the Soy Zone without feeling deprived, hungry, or fatigued. This is because you will gain control over your blood sugar levels and ensure that your brain is given a steady supply of glucose as a fuel source. Furthermore, you will not feel deprived because each of the meals contains large volumes of food. In fact, you may even find that you're eating a greater quantity of food than before.

RULE #4: ADJUST THE SOY ZONE TO YOUR OWN EATING PREFERENCES

If you are a vegan (who eats no animal protein, milk, or dairy products), you will consume practically all of your protein in the form of soy protein. You'll probably need to include processed soy products (like soy meat substitutes or isolated soy protein powders) as a part of every meal to make sure you're getting enough protein. You'll be consuming about 75 grams of soy protein a day if you are a woman, and 100 grams of soy protein a day if you're a man. These are about the same levels of soy protein that the Okinawans consume.

If you're not a vegan (and only 2 percent of all vegetarians are), you can be a little more flexible and include other forms of protein in your Soy Zone Diet. Try to consume at least half your daily protein intake in the form of soy protein. This means about 40 grams of soy protein per day for the average female and 50 grams of soy protein per day for the average male. You can mix and match vegetarian Zone meals with Soy Zone meals. For instance, if you're a lacto-ovo vegetarian, you could have a vegetable omelet made with egg whites for breakfast (a vegetarian Zone meal), a mixed green salad topped with low-fat cottage cheese and orange slices for lunch (another vegetarian Zone meal), and two soy veggie burgers topped with melted soy cheese, steamed vegetables, and fruit for dessert for dinner (a Soy Zone meal).

Finally, if you're not a vegetarian, you can incorporate low-fat animal sources such as fish, poultry, and very lean cuts of beef into your Zone meals, so that you can switch back and forth between Zone meals and Soy Zone meals. In fact, I recommend having at least two to three fish meals (preferably salmon, tuna, or other dark-fleshed fish) per week to get a heart-healthy dose of long-chain Omega-3 fatty acids. To get the full brain-boosting benefits of these fatty acids, you would need to eat at least one fish meal per day or to take an Omega-3 fatty acid supplement.

Regardless of how you mix and match your Soy Zone and Zone meals, follow this rule of thumb: Have either two Soy Zone meals or at least one Soy Zone meal and two Soy Zone snacks every day. Your other meals and snacks should, of course, be Zone-friendly.

RULE #5: YOU'RE ONLY AS HORMONALLY GOOD AS YOUR LAST MEAL

The key to success with the Soy Zone Diet is balancing protein and carbohydrate at *every* meal. Eating virtually all your protein at one meal and then eating virtually all your carbohydrate at the next won't do it. The balance of protein to carbohydrate in each meal and snack determines the hormonal response (good or bad) for the next four to six hours. This is why I say that you're only as hormonally good as your last meal. On the flip side, you can turn your lagging energy from a poor meal around by eating a Zone–friendly meal or snack. Think of it as taking a drug. If you take the right dosage at the right time, the drug works. Following the Soy Zone Diet, you treat your food with the same respect that you would treat any prescription drug.

Realize, too, that if you make a mistake, you haven't lost the battle. You've only left the Zone temporarily, and you can get right back in it at your next meal. That's why there's no guilt on the Soy Zone Diet. In fact, I strongly encourage everyone to eat a high-density carbohydrate meal (like pasta) every month. I want you to experience what an insulin hangover feels like, with the resulting bloating, physical fatigue, and lack of mental focus. This will reinforce what a powerful drug food really is.

Every Soy Zone meal is based on the balance of protein and carbohydrate with a dash of fat. If you follow the eyeball method described in this chapter, you will create the right balance of protein and carbohydrate virtually every time you eat, which will maintain insulin in the appropriate zone. Actually, as I will explain in Chapter 10, there is a little more science than simply eyeballing your portion sizes, but this simple method works for the vast majority of people.

RULE #6: DON'T GO TOO LONG WITHOUT EATING

This may sound impossible, given the fact that you're eating fewer calories than before you went on the Soy Zone. Trust me, though, you may not feel hungry at the time that you need to eat your next meal or snack. In fact, that's how you stay in the Zone: You always eat before you feel too hungry. You know what being famished can do to you, right? You become so ravenous that your stomach feels like a bottomless pit that can never be filled. That feeling is the result of depleted blood sugar for the brain caused by too much insulin coursing through your veins. The lack of blood sugar *is* sending a signal to your brain that you need to eat carbohydrates and lots of them. The key is to eat before your blood sugar levels dip too low, so that you won't be as likely to overeat.

Therefore, the final rule about the Soy Zone Diet: Try to eat five times a day (three meals and two snacks), and never let more than five waking hours go by without eating a Soy Zone meal or snack. A Soy Zone meal should give you a minimum of four to six hours in the Zone, and a Soy Zone snack will give you two to three hours in the Zone. Therefore, just as you plan your daily schedule with regards to appointments, meetings, and even taking medication, also schedule your Zone meals accordingly. A typical schedule might be as follows: if you wake up at 6:00, then eat a Soy Zone breakfast by 7:00. Five hours later, it's noon, and time for lunch, which will be another big meal. Most people don't eat dinner before 7:00, which is more than five hours after lunch, so you must have a snack in the late afternoon. After eating dinner at 7:00, make sure you have one final late-night snack as a hormonal touchup before you go to bed. This will help keep your insulin and blood sugar levels on an even keel until morning. That's a typical day in the Soy Zone (see table on page 24).

Timing of Zone Meals		
Meal	**Timing**	**Approximate Time of the Day**
Breakfast	Within 1 hour after waking	7:00 A.M.
Lunch	Within 5 hours after breakfast	12:00 P.M.
Afternoon Snack	Within 5 hours after lunch	5:00 P.M.
Dinner	Within 2 to 3 hours after snack	7:00 P.M.
Late-night snack	Before bed	11:00 P.M.

How Much Protein Do You Need?

That's the million-dollar question, because protein is the basis of life. Your muscles, your immune system, and every enzyme (the molecular factories that make your body work) are composed of protein. You use up protein every day, which means you must consume adequate amounts of protein to keep your body supplied with this critical nutrient. If you eat too little protein, you can inadvertently begin to shut down all of your body's functions that rely on protein. You lose muscle strength, weaken your body's ability to fight off disease, and, most importantly, decrease your lifespan.

Although protein is critical for life, you should never consume *more* protein than your body requires. On the other hand, consuming *less* than your body needs is equivalent to protein malnutrition. How much protein should you eat each day? Until recently, nutrition experts thought you should eat as little as possible—just enough to avoid overt protein deficiency.

New research, however, challenges this conventional nutritional advice. A study from Harvard Medical School has shown that the more protein women consume, the less likely they are to develop heart disease (the number-one killer of women). The same results probably also apply to men. A second study found that the more protein women consume, the fewer hip fractures they suffer. Still other research suggests that increasing your intake of protein increases the loss of excess body fat. Researchers have also concluded that eating more protein increases a breast cancer patient's chance of survival. With all of this new information, it's now quite clear that consuming more protein leads to better health.

So how can you consume adequate levels of protein without consuming too much? A good rule of thumb is this: Never eat any more low-fat protein at a meal than you can fit in the palm of your hand. Also, make sure it is no thicker than your palm. Based on this advice, then, the average American female needs about 20 grams of protein at a meal, whereas the average American male needs about 30 grams of protein at a meal.

If you are eating three Zone meals and two Zone snacks (each containing about 7 grams of protein), this amounts to about 75 grams of protein per day for the average woman, and 100 grams per day for the average male. This may seem like a lot of protein, but it's actually very similar to the protein levels that most Americans presently consume (although they are consuming far more carbohydrates than recommended on the Soy Zone). Keep in mind, too, that the Okinawans consume more than 100 grams of protein per day, and look at what this has done for them!

Not everyone, though, has the same exact protein requirements. If you are considerably overweight or a highly trained athlete, you will actually need more protein than the average individual. In Chapter 7, I will show you how to calculate your exact protein prescription. For the vast majority of Americans, however, the levels of protein consumption described above are sufficient to meet their bodies' needs and provide the health benefits cited in the latest medical research.

SOY ZONE SUPPLEMENTS

On the Soy Zone Diet, you're consuming a bountiful supply of fruits and vegetables, which are rich in vitamins and minerals. Fruits and vegetables contain far more of these micronutrients than high-density carbohydrates like grains and starches. In fact, pasta, bread, and rice are pretty poor sources of vitamins and minerals. In a ranking, vegetables would come out on top, with fruits coming in second and grains a distant third. Just compare the nutrients found in specific foods from these categories in the table below.

Comparison of Vitamin and Mineral Content of Various Carbohydrates (Serving 10 Grams of Carbohydrates)							
Carbohydrate	Amount	Vitamin A	Vitamin C	Folic Acid	Magnesium	Calcium	Fiber
Broccoli	3 cups	6,492	348	234	114	210	13.2
Kiwi	1	133	57	1.0	23	19	2.5
Rice, brown	⅕ cup	0	0	1.6	21	0.9	0.7

Given the fact that you'll be meeting most of your vitamin and mineral needs through the Soy Zone, you don't need to take a multivitamin/mineral supplement. (You can if you want to, as a form of cheap insurance, but you probably don't need it.) There are, however, three vital nutrients that may be lacking on any diet, including the Soy Zone. I strongly urge you to take a daily dose of a long-chain Omega-3 fatty acid supplement, a vitamin E supplement, and a vitamin B_{12} supplement—especially if you are a vegan.

LONG-CHAIN OMEGA-3 FATTY ACIDS

Unless you are eating one or two fish meals a day, you're probably not getting enough long-chain Omega-3 fatty acids. These fatty acids are critical for maintaining optimal performance in your brain, your cardiovascular system, and your immune system. Without realizing it, your grandmother recognized the importance of these fatty acids when she made your parents take cod liver oil. Cod liver oil is without a doubt one of the world's worst-tasting items, but it contains high levels of long-chain Omega-3 fatty acids.

One type of Omega-3 fatty acid is called docosahexanenoic acid (DHA). DHA is found throughout the fatty tissue in your brain, and it appears to play a role in how your brain functions. A growing body of research has confirmed that infants who are deficient in levels of this fatty acid have less than optimal neurological responses, especially intelligence. Furthermore, a great number of neurological conditions, such as depression, attention deficit disorder, and schizophrenia, also have a high correlation with deficient levels of DHA in the bloodstream. More conclusively, researchers have found that patients with bipolar depression (the most difficult form of depression to treat) often respond dramatically to very high-dose supplementation with oils rich in DHA.

You can get adequate amounts of DHA by eating one serving a day of a fish rich in Omega-3 fatty acids. These are generally the darker-fleshed fish like salmon, tuna, and mackerel. You can also take fish oil supplements to ensure that you are getting enough. If you're a vegetarian, a new option is available for DHA supplementation: Scientists have developed certain algae that produce a large amount of DHA-containing oils. Supplements using these DHA-rich oils solve the problem of getting enough DHA for optimal brain function for the vegetarian.

My recommendation:
I recommend about 5 to 10 grams per day of fish oil supplements in soft gelatin capsules (only about one-third of the oil in the capsule is actually composed of long-chain Omega-3 fatty acids). If you are a vegetarian or don't consume any fish products, you can take 1 to 3 grams a day of algae oil supplements in capsule form. Consuming 5 to 10 capsules per day may seem like a lot, but it's actually less than the amount of long-chain Omega-3 fatty acids contained in the tablespoon of cod liver oil that your grandmother served up.

VITAMIN E

Regardless of whether or not you're a vegetarian, you're probably not consuming enough vitamin E to reap its full benefits. The richest source of vitamin E is vegetable oil, which is used in moderation on the Soy Zone. Vitamin E is an antioxidant, meaning it destroys deadly substances called *free radicals* that can destroy healthy cells or turn them cancerous. A vast body of research has found that people who take vitamin E supplements have lower rates of heart disease. The scientific data overwhelmingly supports the increased intake of vitamin E in every diet.

Although the RDA for vitamin E is 10 international units (IU) for males and 8 IU for females, all the available clinical studies indicate that optimal health benefits from this vitamin only occur when vitamin E intake is greater than 100 IU per day. My recommendation: You should take 400 IU per day to ensure that you reap the maximum health benefits of vitamin E.

VITAMIN B$_{12}$

If you're a vegan or lacto-ovo vegetarian, you should probably also supplement your Soy Zone Diet with vitamin B$_{12}$. This vitamin helps maintain the production of red blood cells in the bone marrow and helps maintain the normal functioning of your nervous system. This vitamin is found primarily in beef, chicken, and pork, though it's found in lower amounts in egg and dairy products. Vegans are more likely to be deficient in vitamin B$_{12}$. A deficiency can cause extreme fatigue and depression. My recommendation: Unfortunately, supplements of vitamin B$_{12}$ aren't well absorbed by the body, so you'll need to take about 50 micrograms per day in order to get the recommended dosage of 2 micrograms that you would naturally ingest from eating animal protein.

So there you have it: Your basic road map to the Soy Zone. Follow the rules I outlined in this chapter and supplement your diet with long-chain Omega-3 fatty acids and vitamin E. If you're a vegetarian, consider a vitamin B$_{12}$ supplement as well. If you find that you're not eating a wide variety of vegetables (especially green leafy ones) and fruits, take a multivitamin/mineral capsule every day as a cheap insurance policy. Keep in mind, though, that taking megadoses of vitamins and minerals won't overcome a hormonally poor diet that's created by eating excessive amounts of carbohydrates. Put your efforts into preparing and enjoying Soy Zone meals, not taking massive amounts of supplements.

Now that you know the rules for getting into and staying in the Zone, let's look at the practical ways to implement them. It's time to give your kitchen a makeover. When you're through with the next chapter, your kitchen will be fully equipped and Soy Zone–friendly.

3

Zoning Your Kitchen

Let's face it: Most of us aren't going to make any dietary change unless it's easy. We live in a fast-paced, deadline-driven world, and we simply don't have the time to spend hours in the kitchen preparing complicated dishes for every meal. I kept this in mind when I created the Soy Zone. I knew that this plan had to be simple and easy to implement. Don't worry if you've never cooked a vegetarian meal in your life—or any meal, for that matter. Chapters 4 and 5 tell you everything you need to know to make Soy Zone meals in minutes. First, though, you need to get your kitchen ready for action.

WHAT TO TOSS OUT

Your first step is to create shelf space by tossing out (or sealing away in a box in your basement) all high-density carbohydrates, such as pasta, rice, and bread that have been major staples in your diet. I'm not saying that you'll never eat these foods again. You can—in much greater moderation—but I want you to try to abstain from eating them for a few weeks to give yourself time to get used to being on the Soy Zone. After you feel like you've got the plan down, you can add these items back in, in small amounts. In fact, I want you to think of them as condiments, rather than as side dishes or (even worse!) the main course. Getting rid of these foods will not only remove temptations from your kitchen while you're learning the basics of the Soy Zone Diet, but will create space for all the Soy Zone–friendly foods that you'll be stocking in your kitchen. Here is a list of food items that you need to banish (at least temporarily) from your kitchen:

FOODS TO REMOVE FROM YOUR KITCHEN

- White and brown rice

- Pasta

- Breakfast cereals and cereal-based nutrition bars

- Instant mashed potato

- Polenta, couscous, bulgur wheat, and other grains (except barley and steel-cut oatmeal)

- Bread (including whole wheat and whole grain), breadsticks, and tortillas

- Ice cream, sorbet, tofu ice cream, and Popsicles

- Potato chips, corn chips, pretzels, and crackers

- Cake, cookies, and other sweets

- White and whole wheat flour

- Cornstarch

- Sugar

- Juice (including orange juice and apple juice)

- Sugary sodas

- Sweetened yogurt

- Honey

FOODS TO STOCK IN YOUR KITCHEN

Now that you have a lot more space, stock your pantry and refrigerator full of the new staples that will help you prepare balanced Soy Zone meals quickly and easily. I've divided this section into soy proteins, carbohydrates, and fats. In each category, I describe my favorite foods and give you some advice on where to find them, how to prepare them, and where to store them.

PROTEIN

Protein is the most crucial element on the Soy Zone Diet, and at least half of your daily intake should consist of soy protein products. You need to get adequate amounts of this protein at each meal and snack—especially if you are a vegan and don't eat protein from animal sources. As I already discussed, soybean protein can result in an even more improved control of your insulin levels compared to animal protein. Regardless of your current dietary habits, I believe that by the time you finish reading this book you will dramatically increase your consumption of soy protein products.

When choosing between soy products, realize that not all soy is created equal as far as the protein content is concerned. Many traditional soy products, such as boiled soybeans, soy milk, and some forms of tempeh, also contain significant amounts of carbohydrates in addition to protein. Like cow's milk and natural yogurt, these products contain a *good* ratio of protein to carbohydrates. You can eat them by themselves as a snack or meal, but if you add in some fruits or vegetables you may wind up consuming too many carbohydrates, which can send you out of the Zone.

Only the more processed forms of soybeans, such as tofu, soy meat substitutes, and soy protein isolates, are very rich in protein and relatively poor in carbohydrates. My advice? Scan the food labels of all the soy products you purchase to see how many grams of protein and how many grams of carbohydrate each serving contains. In order to qualify as a protein serving, a soy product should contain *at least* twice as much protein as carbohydrate. If the product contains less protein, you can't use it as a protein source that you can combine with carbohydrates. Think of it, instead, as a stand-alone meal or as a Soy Zone snack.

SOY PROTEIN TO USE FOR YOUR MEALS

Meat Substitutes

Meat alternatives, made from soybeans, contain soy protein or tofu and other ingredients mixed together to look and taste like various kinds of meat. These meat alternatives are sold as frozen, canned, or dried foods. Usually they can be used the same way as the foods they replace. With so many different meat alternatives available to consumers, the nutritional value of these foods varies considerably. Usually they are lower in fat, but check the label to be sure. Here are a few specific ones:

Soy Hamburger Crumbles

I consider this the biggest breakthrough in soybean processing technology. This soybean product looks and tastes like ground hamburger. Many dishes that use ground hamburger can be reproduced with this product. It is incredibly easy to use because it can be taken directly from the freezer or refrigerator to the skillet. It also takes on spices and flavorings very readily. Many recipes in Chapter 5 contain soy hamburger crumbles, which can be found in supermarkets as well as natural food stores. The brand that I prefer is Harvest Burger-Style Recipe Crumbles, made by Morningstar Farms.

Soy Burgers

The newest soybean hamburgers are extremely tasty. My personal favorite is a brand called Boca Burger, because it has a good balance of protein to carbohydrate (although not as favorable as the soy hamburger crumbles), and the burgers are individually wrapped to minimize freezer burn. Read the label carefully, since many soy burgers contain almost pure carbohydrate.

Soy Sausages and Hot Dogs

Soy sausage links are great for breakfast because they tend to be spicier than other soy products. Soy hot dogs have come a great distance, but frankly (no pun intended), they still need to beef up their taste. Add some mustard and relish to achieve a closer version of a real hot dog.

Soy Deli Meats

Soy salami, bologna, and turkey slices are worth trying. They still need more tinkering, though, before they put the deli counter at the supermarket out of business.

SOY FLOUR

Soy flour is made from roasted soybeans ground into a fine powder. There are three kinds of soy flour available: **Natural or full-fat** contains the natural oils found in the soybean; however, the high oil content can cause it to go rancid in a short period of time. **Defatted** has the oils removed during processing, which makes it more stable for storage. **Lecithinated** soy flour has had soy lecithin added to it to give it better mixing characteristics. Soy flour can be used for a variety of cooking baking purposes to give a protein boost to recipes. Since it doesn't contain any gluten (which wheat does), however, you can only use small amounts of it, or the product won't rise.

SOY GRITS

These are dry soybeans that have been lightly toasted and then cracked in small pieces. Soy grits can be used as a substitute for flour in some recipes. They can also be used as an additive to sauces to increase their protein content.

SOY PROTEIN POWDERS

The type of isolated soy protein powder that I recommend is known as *soy protein isolates.* Soy protein isolates, the most highly refined soy protein, contain more than 90 percent protein. Soy concentrates, another form of soy protein powder, have a slightly lower protein concentration (about 70 percent). Soy protein powders can be added to virtually any food (like dips, oatmeal, fruit smoothies, etc.) to increase the protein-to-carbohydrate balance. In addition, they are shelf-stable, so no refrigeration is required.

Note: Lacto-ovo vegetarians and non-vegetarians may choose from a greater variety of protein powders. One especially popular form is deionized whey protein powder, a by-product of cheese production, which tends to taste better than soybean isolates. It also, however, produces a greater insulin stimulation than soy protein isolates. Therefore, you should try mixing both products together until you get the best taste using the most amount of soy protein isolates. As with all soy protein powders, isolated protein powders from egg or milk can be stored at room temperature, always ensuring easy access to protein to fortify any meal.

TEMPEH

Tempeh originated in Indonesia and is made of hulled, cooked soybeans (or soybeans mixed with grains or seeds) that are fermented with a mold until they form a chunky, tender soybean cake. Tempeh is more easily digested than other traditional soy foods. It can be marinated and grilled and added to soups, casseroles, or chili. Since raw tempeh soaks up oil at an astonishing rate, for best results brush each piece very lightly with oil and brown in a nonstick skillet.

Tempeh is typically sold in 8-ounce or 16-ounce vacuum-wrapped slabs, either refrigerated or frozen. You can find it in Asian or natural food stores. Don't be concerned if you notice any gray or blackish spots on the surface, which is simply the mold used to make tempeh that can be cut away before the tempeh is cooked.

Tempeh comes in many varieties, depending upon what additional ingredients are combined with the soybeans. Pure soy tempeh has the strongest taste, while mixed-grain tempehs are a better choice for more delicate preparations and for newcomers to this tasty food. However, be careful to read the label of tempeh products carefully, because mixed-grain tempeh will contain higher amounts of carbohydrate that may make it unsuitable as a protein-rich source on the Soy Zone Diet.

TEXTURED SOY PROTEIN

Textured soy protein is made from defatted soy flour and has a chewy texture. To make this product, defatted soy flour is cooked in water under high pressure, and then passed through an extruder under pressure. As it passes through the die at the end of the extruder, different sizes and shapes of granules can be made. These granules are then dried to form textured soy protein.

To prepare textured soy protein granules for cooking, you have to hydrate them in boiling water and then drain off any excess water before using. The product is marketed by Archer Daniels Midland under the name Textured Vegetable Protein (TVP). TVP takes a lot of preparation time and has a higher carbohydrate content than other soy products. I would advise sticking with the newer soy products for better taste.

TOFU

Tofu is the king of traditional soy products. It is protein-rich and extremely versatile, making it ideal to balance carbohydrates for Soy Zone meals. Tofu, also known as soybean curd, is a soft cheese-like food made by curdling fresh hot soy milk with a coagulant. Depending upon how much liquid is extracted from the curds, the tofu is labeled as soft, medium, firm, or extra-firm. *The firmer the tofu, the more protein it contains relative to carbohydrate.* Silken tofu is a creamy product and can be used as a replacement for sour cream in many dip recipes. It does, though, contain more carbohydrates and less protein than firm tofu.

Fresh Chinese-style organic tofu is readily available in vacuum-packed one-pound blocks in refrigerated tubs. Sealed, refrigerated tofu is a better choice than the small squares of tofu that you'll find soaking in water at room temperature in Asian grocery stores. These are open to air and possible contamination and usually are not made from organic soybeans.

When purchasing tofu, note the expiration date. (If the expiration date will pass before you've had a chance to cook it, pop the unopened tub into the freezer and follow the instructions that I'll provide later for cooking frozen tofu.) Once you've opened the container, refrigerate any leftovers in water in a tightly sealed container. Change the water every day or so and the tofu will remain fresh for about five days. The scent of fresh tofu is faintly sweet and slightly beany. Like any fresh food, tofu can breed bacteria and should always be handled with care and clean hands. If you detect a sour smell or the tofu becomes dark around the edges, discard it.

Tofu is like the chicken of the vegetable kingdom: It has a mild taste and readily takes on a wide variety of flavors. To maximize taste and texture, there are several things you should keep in mind. First of all, what type? Firm and extra-firm Chinese-style fresh tofu is the best choice for stir-fries, kebobs, cutlets, or any other dish that requires tofu to have optimum taste and hold its shape. Silken Japanese-style tofu is a convenient choice for making dips, dressings, vegetable purees, and smoothies.

Hints for Preparing and Storing Tofu

Draining: You should drain tofu before using by removing it from the water and setting it in a strainer.

Pressing: If you're using firm or extra-firm tofu, you may want to press it to make it firmer and avoid ending up with a watery stir-fry or stew. Pressed tofu also becomes more sponge-like and absorbs flavor more effectively. The simplest way to press tofu is to loosely wrap the block in several layers of a clean kitchen towel and set a heavy pan on top. Let the tofu sit for at least 15 minutes.

Freezing: You can freeze an unopened tub of tofu until you are ready to use it. Don't freeze silken tofu, though, because you can ruin its texture. To defrost frozen tofu quickly, puncture the top of the tub a dozen times, set on a lidded plate, and defrost in a microwave for five to seven minutes. Alternatively, defrost at room temperature, which will take about three hours. Drain the tofu and press it firmly between two plates to extract all of the liquid. Tofu that has been frozen is a few shades darker than fresh, has a delightfully chewy texture, and absorbs flavor like a sponge. It's a highly recommended way to give tofu a completely different taste.

SOY SNACKS

Boiled Green Soybeans

Although there are hundreds of varieties of soybeans, the three main types are green, beige, and black. Fresh green soybeans are those harvested when they're still young and sweet-tasting and can be served as a snack or a main vegetable dish. Boil them in slightly salted water for 15 to 20 minutes and serve straight from their pods. Kept in the refrigerator, they are also great snacks. Fresh or frozen green soybeans are sold in Asian and natural food stores, shelled or still in the pod. Beige and black soybeans are sold either dried or cooked and canned. Good-quality organic soybeans are also available in ready-to-eat cans.

Soy Cheese and Yogurt

These products are made from soy milk. They have a creamy texture, making it easy to substitute them for sour cream or cream cheese and can be found in a variety of flavors in natural foods stores. Products made with soy cheese include soy pizza, and you can also make soy cheeseburgers. Soy cheeses are available as either a hard cheese or cream cheese. With soy yogurts, read the label carefully, since many manufacturers will add extra carbohydrates like sugar to improve the taste—just like they do for regular yogurt.

Soy Health Bars

Ever since the U.S. government stated that any food product that contains at least 6.25 grams of soy protein can be declared "heart-healthy," more and more candy bars are being reformulated with soy protein to be "heart-healthy" candy bars. Look carefully at the label. If the bar contains twice as many carbohydrates compared to protein, then it's still a candy bar that will cause a rise in insulin levels—not so heart-healthy after all.

Soy Milk

Soy milk is made from ground soybeans that are simmered in water and strained, then pressed to extract the nutrient-rich beige liquid. Soy milk is sold in boxes that can be stored at room temperature until they are opened, but be sure to use them before the expiration date marked on the package. Opened containers will last for a week to ten days in the refrigerator. Soy milk is also sold as a powder, which must be mixed with water.

When shopping for soy milk, it's wise to check the labels and compare brands, as manufacturers may add a wide range of sweeteners and other ingredients, often extra carbohydrates, to enhance its appeal to the American palate. These extra carbohydrates eliminate the benefit of the natural balance of protein and carbohydrate in these soy products. Packaged soy milk can be found in most supermarkets and health food stores

Fresh soy milk has a milder taste and less body than shelf-stable soy milk. Of course, it has none of the added ingredients common to aseptic-packed brands. It is quite delicious as a morning drink, especially for those accustomed to skim milk.

You can make your own soy milk quite inexpensively in one of the electric soy milk makers now on the market. Salton makes an efficient and reasonably priced model that can be found in many large houseware stores.

Soy Nuts

These are soy equivalent of peanuts, and they make a great Soy Zone snack by themselves. You can find them at natural food stores. You also can make them yourself by soaking soybeans for about 3 hours. Place them on an oiled cookie sheet and bake at 350 degrees and turn them every few minutes until they are well browned.

SOY CONDIMENTS

Soy Sauces

Miso

Miso is a rich, salty condiment that characterizes the essence of Japanese cooking. A smooth paste, miso is made from cooked soybeans, grains, salt, and a mold culture and then aged in cedar vats for one to three years. It should be refrigerated. Use miso to flavor soups, sauces, dressings, marinades, and pâtés. You can buy miso in Asian markets.

Natto

Natto is made of fermented, cooked whole soybeans. Because the fermentation process breaks down the beans' complex proteins, natto is more easily digested than whole soybeans. It has a sticky, viscous coating with a cheesy texture. In Asian countries, natto traditionally is served as a topping for rice, in miso soups, or stirred into vegetables. It can be found in Asian and natural food stores.

Shoyu

This is the true soy sauce that is used in the Far East. Like miso, shoyu is made by combining cooked soybeans, a grain, and a mold culture in a salty brine for 12 to 18 months. The soy sauce that most Americans are familiar with is a product composed of defatted soybean meal and wheat mixed with chemicals. Add a little caramel coloring and corn syrup and within a few days you have a soy sauce that has a very inferior taste to shoyu.

Tamari

This is liquid left over from the fermentation of miso. It can be used as a form of shoyu.

SOY FIBER

There are two basic types of soy fiber: Okara and soy bran. All of these products are high-quality, inexpensive sources of dietary fiber, and they can all be found in natural food stores. **Okara** is a pulp fiber by-product of soymilk. It has less protein than whole soybeans, but the protein remaining is of high quality. Okara tastes similar to coconut and can be baked or added as fiber to granola and cookies. It is very perishable, though, and must be used within a few days even if refrigerated. **Soy bran** is made from the hulls (outer covering) of the soybean. The hulls contain a fibrous material that can be extracted and then refined for use as a food ingredient.

Soy Sprouts

Although not as popular as mung bean sprouts or alfalfa sprouts, soy sprouts (also called soybean sprouts) are an excellent source of nutrition, packed with more protein and Vitamin C than typical sprouts. They can be sprouted in the same manner as other beans and seeds. Soy sprouts must be cooked quickly at low heat so that they don't get mushy. They can also be used raw in salads or soups, or in stir-fried, sautéed, or baked dishes.

Yuba

When soy milk is warmed, the skin that forms at the top is yuba. It can then be dried and made into sheets, which, after it has been soaked in water, can be used to wrap vegetables. Dried yuba sheets (called dried bean curd, bean curd sheets, or bean curd skin) can be found in Asian food stores.

CARBOHYDRATES

Now that you've stocked your kitchen with a wide variety of soy protein products, you're ready to stock up on carbohydrates (low-density ones, of course) to balance your Soy Zone meal. Since your goal is to keep your insulin levels within the Zone, you should consume primarily vegetables supplemented with fruits—with very few starches and grains. Even with fruits and vegetables, you have to be somewhat careful in your choices: Some fruits (such as bananas and watermelons) and some vegetables (such as carrots and corn) enter the bloodstream very rapidly, which increases insulin levels more quickly than other fruits and vegeta-

bles. (See Appendix D for the most favorable types of fruits and vegetables for making Soy Zone meals.)

When choosing fruits and vegetables, aim for a variety in a rainbow
of colors. The colors are indicative of a wide variety of phytochemicals
and antioxidants that can be useful in conjunction with the Soy Zone
Diet to reduce the risk of certain diseases, such as heart disease and cancer. The best choices for fruit include apples, apricots, pears, oranges,
raspberries, plums, kiwi, blueberries, strawberries, grapes, and grapefruit. The best choices for vegetables include dark green leafy vegetables,
broccoli, cauliflower, tomatoes, mushrooms, and peppers.

You have three options for stocking your kitchen with fruits and
vegetables. The first is to go to the supermarket two or three times a
week to get fresh produce. These food items don't last long, so don't
make the mistake of overbuying and then getting stuck with rotten produce. To avoid a lot of cutting and peeling, think about purchasing
bagged, precut and prepeeled vegetables and fruits twice a week. Or get
all the precut produce you need from the supermarket salad bar.

Your second option is to use frozen fruits and vegetables. They last
longer, prevent the need for frequent shopping, are less expensive, and take
little time to prepare. Fortunately, advances in food technology are also
making frozen vegetables and fruits taste far better than in the past. You
may also be surprised to learn that frozen vegetables and fruits are *more*
nutritious than many fresh vegetables because they are frozen almost
immediately after harvesting, thus preserving much of their nutrient content. On the other hand, fresh vegetables and fruits may be several weeks
old before they reach your refrigerator and can lose much of their vitamin
content during their journey from the orchard to your plate.

Your third option, which I consider the least desirable one by far, is
to purchase canned vegetables and fruits. Although canned produce is
cheaper than fresh or frozen, it has a much lower vitamin and mineral
content (except for excessive salt) than fresh or frozen items. You can
add sauces and seasonings to improve the taste of canned produce. If
you eat canned produce regularly, you should consider taking a vitamin
and mineral supplement to compensate for the lower amount of vitamins and minerals.

Should You Buy Organic Produce?

If you're concerned about the contamination of produce by pesticides and herbicides (which should be a legitimate concern), then purchase organic items. Be prepared, however, to pay a higher price and have a more limited selection. If organic vegetables are not readily available, here are some helpful hints to minimize any potential contamination concerns:

1. Peel off the outer skin with a peeler if possible.

2. If the fruit or vegetable can't be peeled, scrub the outer surface with a vegetable brush and then rinse under cold water.

3. For vegetables such as lettuce, discard the outer leaves, and wash the remaining leaves.

4. For berries or other items that can't be peeled, rinse with cold water several times.

FATS

On the Soy Zone Diet, you should focus on eating primarily monounsaturated fats while reducing your intake of unhealthy fats. These unhealthy fats include saturated fats (found in butter, whole milk, full-fat dairy products, and red meat) and trans fatty acids (found in margarine and partially hydrogenated oils) because both of these are known to increase cholesterol levels and the risk of heart disease. In addition, oils containing high levels of Omega-6 fatty acids (soybean, safflower, sunflower, and corn oils) should be avoided. Excess levels of Omega-6 fats can eliminate many of the benefits of the Soy Zone Diet because they cause the overproduction of a group of hormones called *eicosanoids*, which can have damaging effects on the body. (I explain these hormones in greater detail in my books *The Zone* and *The Anti-Aging Zone*.)

The primary oil you should use for sautéing and baking is refined olive oil, which is less expensive and more resistant to oxidation during cooking (oxidation increases free radical production) than virgin olive oil. Sesame oil is another good option for cooking because it is also very resistant to oxidation. You can use both canola oil and extra-virgin olive oil (both high in monounsaturated fats) for salad dressings since they won't oxidize if they aren't heated. Other oils rich in monounsaturated fats include those made from macadamia, almond, and cashew nuts.

Store opened bottles of oil in a dark pantry. Exposing oils to light can reduce their shelf life. Oils generally have a four-month shelf life, so purchase them in small amounts. The following table gives a listing of the appropriate oils for your Soy Zone kitchen.

Preferred Oils for the Soy Zone

Best for Cooking

> Refined olive oil
>
> Sesame oil

Best for Salad Dressings

> Canola oil
>
> Extra-virgin olive oil

Avoid (rich in Omega-6 fatty acids)

> Soybean oil
>
> Sunflower oil
>
> Safflower oil
>
> Corn oil

Soy Lecithin

This is the phospholipid fraction extracted from soybean oil. Lecithin is used in food manufacturing as an emulsifing agent for products high in fats and oils and can replace egg yolks (which are also rich in lecithin). Food-grade lecithin is usually in the form of thick viscous liquid containing residual soybean oil; however, defatted lecithin can be found in natural health food stores.

Soybean Oil

Ironically, this is the only part of the soybean that I don't like. Soybean oil is naturally extracted from whole soybeans. It is the most widely used oil in the United States, often sold in the grocery store under the generic name "vegetable oil." Soybean oil contains high levels of unhealthy Omega-6 fatty acids, which is why I don't recommend using this oil.

OTHER FOOD STAPLES FOR THE SOY ZONE KITCHEN

Although fruits and vegetables will be your primary source of carbohydrates on the Soy Zone Diet, they don't have to be your sole sources. You can include other kinds of carbohydrates, but eat only moderate amounts of them because they contain a higher density of carbohydrates. Here are some examples.

Beans and Legumes

These represent one of my favorite Soy Zone items because of their high content of soluble fiber, which helps slow the rate of carbohydrate entry into the bloodstream, thus reducing insulin secretion. They also contain relatively more protein than other vegetable items. Unfortunately, only 70 percent of the stated protein on the label will actually be absorbed by your body, because a good deal of the protein passes through your system bound to the indigestible fiber found in beans and legumes. What's more, since beans and legumes (except soybeans) contain larger amounts of carbohydrates relative to their protein content, they can't be used with wild abandon if your goal is to control your insulin levels. The table below shows you how various beans compare when it comes to their content of carbohydrates and absorbable protein.

Protein and Carbohydrate Composition of Various Volumes of Boiled Beans		
	Protein Grams	**Carbohydrate Grams**
Chickpeas (2/3 cup)	7	27
Black beans (2/3 cup)	7	18
Lentils (1/2 cup)	7	13
Navy beans (2/3 cup)	7	27
Pinto beans (2/3 cup)	7	18
Red kidney beans (2/3 cup)	7	18
Soybeans (1/3 cup)	7	6

As you can also see, only soybeans contain more protein than carbohydrate. In fact, most beans (other than lentils) contain relatively massive amounts of carbohydrates compared to protein. Therefore, treat most beans (other than soybeans) primarily as a carbohydrate source rather than a protein source. If you're eating beans, fill one-third of your plate with a protein-rich soy protein and one-third of the plate with beans. Leave the rest of your plate empty or fill it with mixed greens (which contain very small amounts of carbohydrates).

Oatmeal and Barley

Use most grains as condiments on the Soy Zone because of their high carbohydrate density. The two grains that I prefer are oatmeal (slow-cooking types such as steel-cut or Irish oatmeal) and barley. Both are rich in soluble fiber, which slows down their entry rate into the bloodstream, causing a smaller surge in insulin. Both have a long shelf life if kept in tightly sealed containers away from light. Nonetheless, both are still very carbohydrate-dense, so you must be careful not to overconsume them.

Nuts and Nut Butters

Although nuts contain some protein, they are primarily a source of fat. Try to choose nuts that are particularly rich in monounsaturated fats. The best source is macadamia nuts; other sources include almonds, pistachios, hazelnuts, and cashews. Not surprisingly, the more expensive the nut, the higher its monounsaturated fat content. The best nut butter is almond butter because of its high monounsaturated fat content. Natural peanut butter also contains a plentiful amount of monounsaturated fat, although not nearly as much as almond butter. Soy nut butter is made from roasted whole soy nuts, which are then crushed and blended with soybean oil and other ingredients. Soy nut butter has a slightly nutty taste and significantly less fat than peanut butter. However, since it is rich in Omega-6 fatty acids, I don't recommend it.

Spices

The key to Soy Zone cooking (and any cooking, for that matter) is the use of spices. Each regional cuisine has developed its own unique blend of spices that gives any food a distinctive flavor. The same is true of Soy Zone cooking. Use the right combination of spices, and you instantly create international cuisine. Here are some of the flavorings used for different regional dishes. You'll find many of these spices listed in the Soy Zone recipes.

Chinese: Anise, garlic, and ginger

French: Bay leaves, garlic, rosemary, tarragon, and thyme

Greek: Cinnamon, garlic, mint, and oregano

Indian: Cardamom, coriander seeds, cumin, curry, fenugreek, ginger, mustard seeds, and turmeric

Italian: Basil, bay leaves, fennel seeds, garlic, marjoram, oregano, red pepper flakes, rosemary, and sage

Mexican: Chili, cilantro, cinnamon, cumin, coriander, and oregano

Middle Eastern: Cinnamon, cumin, garlic, mint, parsley, and oregano

Congratulations! You now have a well-stocked Soy Zone kitchen. Before you delve into the recipes in Chapter 5, read the next chapter for some simple and essential cooking tips.

4

Soy Zone
Cooking Tips

Now that your kitchen is stocked with ingredients for Soy Zone meals, you may need some basics to help you develop good cooking skills. Like any craft, cooking requires some special equipment and the mastery of a few basic techniques. If you're already a proficient cook, you can just skim through this chapter. If you feel like you're all thumbs in the kitchen, however, this chapter will tell you which reliable tools you need and how to use them. You may purchase most of the equipment you'll need at a well-stocked kitchen supply store near you, or through a catalogue or over the Internet.

KNIVES

Chefs may argue passionately about the best-tasting olive oil, but none would disagree about the most essential kitchen tool: the chef's knife. Since you'll be chopping a fair amount of fresh vegetables on the Soy Zone Diet, a good chef's knife will quickly become your best friend in the kitchen.

Look for a knife with an 8- or 10-inch blade. Try holding a variety of brands (Henckels and Wusthoff are two fine choices) of both sizes in your hand. Set the blade of each down on a cutting board, and make a chopping motion. Compare for weight and feel, then opt for the knife that is the most comfortable. Carbon-steel knives hold their edges better, but discolor some foods. In addition, you must dry them thoroughly after each use or they will rust. Stainless steel knives require less daily attention, but need to be sharpened more often. Like most things in life, it's a tradeoff.

A small paring knife is not as essential but very useful, especially for coring tomatoes or cutting small fruits and vegetables. An inexpensive medium-sized serrated knife makes slicing tomatoes a breeze.

Chopping is easy and fun when your knife is sharp. On the other hand, a dull knife can be a real hazard, since it forces you to press down very hard, and if the knife slips, you can cut yourself badly. As soon as you sense that your knife has lost its edge, use a sharpening stone and a honing steel or an electric sharpener to get it back into top-notch form.

CUTTING AND CHOPPING

Treat yourself to two spacious cutting boards—one for vegetables and the other for fruit. (You don't want to risk having your kiwi scented with garlic or onions!) Should they be plastic, wood, or hard rubber? Again, it's a tradeoff: Wood is easier on your knife, but plastic is lighter and can be thrown into the dishwasher. If you do opt for plastic, make sure it's the softer kind (due to a lower plastic density) that doesn't damage knives. Generally, the better choice is opaque white rather than clear plastic, but ask a knowledgeable salesperson for advice. If you have access to a restaurant-supply store, you're in luck because the hard rubber chopping mats used in commercial kitchens are the best choice of all.

Once you have your chopping board and a sharp chef's knife ready, hold the knife firmly in your dominant hand and hold the ingredient in place with your other hand—knuckles curled under so that your fingertips are out of view (and therefore out of the knife's range). Use your knuckles to guide the movement of the knife, moving them away as the knife approaches with a rocking up-and-down motion. (Keep the tip of the knife in contact with the board at all times, and rock the blade up and down.) After the ingredient is sliced or coarsely chopped, you may want to mince it into very fine pieces. In this case, hold the tip of the knife to the chopping board with one hand as you rock the knife up and down with the other hand in an arc. When it comes to knife skills, practice really does make perfect, so take heart and let the chopping begin!

Understanding Common Cutting and Chopping Terms

One of the biggest problems for beginning cooks is understanding recipe terminology. Here are definitions for the chopping terms you'll see commonly in recipes:

coarsely chopped: cut into relatively large, irregular pieces

chopped: cut into smallish pieces of irregular shape and size

minced: chopped into very fine, irregular shapes; the term usually refers to preparing fresh garlic, ginger, and potent herbs

diced: cut into small precise cubes, usually about $1/4$ inch (finely diced) or $1/2$ to 1 inches (large dice)

julienned: cut into matchsticks

shredded: chopped into very thin strips, like coleslaw

YOUR PRACTICE RUN

Even if you have the proper knives and know the proper terms, you still need a little practice. Here's a run-through to learn how to properly use your knives.

Chopping an Onion

Onions are one of the workhorses of the Soy Zone kitchen. Most recipes in this book will direct you to chop them, meaning that you can cut them quickly and without precision. Here's how:

1. Cut off the root and stem ends.

2. Slice the onion in half from root to stem (the long way) and peel off the skin.

3. Set the onion cut side down on the chopping board.

4. Slice it thinly lengthwise.

5. Holding the slices together, give the onion a quarter-turn and slice it again at right angles. Discard the small section of the root end that doesn't fall into small pieces.

Dicing an Onion

This technique requires an extra step and produces bits of roughly equal size:

1. Cut off only the stem end, leaving the root intact. Then proceed to steps 2 and 3 above.

2. Make several horizontal cuts ($1/4$ inch thick for fine dice; $1/2$ inch thick for large dice) from stem toward root end.

3. Proceed with steps 4 and 5 above.

Mincing Garlic

1. First peel the individual clove. Loosen the skin, either by pressing the clove firmly under the blade of your chef's knife or by putting the clove inside an E-Z-Rol Garlic Peeler (a clever gadget that is readily available and really works). Then lift off the skin.

2. Slice the clove lengthwise, and if you spot a tiny green shoot running down the middle, remove it, as it can be bitter and hard to digest.

3. Lay the halved clove flat-side down on a chopping board and slice it thinly lengthwise. Then give it a quarter-turn and slice it thinly crosswise.

Quick Tip: If you are using a food processor for the recipe, toss a peeled garlic clove through the feed tube into the bowl while the motor is running.

Dicing Zucchini, Cucumber, and Celery

1. Trim off both ends and peel if necessary.

2. Cut in half lengthwise. Scoop out the seeds from large cucumbers and zucchini.

3. Cut each in half lengthwise again. Hold the long strips together, and cut the thinnest possible slices crosswise.

Chopping and Cleaning Leeks

1. Trim off and discard the tough dark green leaves and root end.

2. Cut small leeks in half and large leeks in quarters lengthwise.

3. Holding the slices together, beginning at root end, cut thin slices crosswise through white and light green parts. Discard any remaining portions of tough, dark leaves.

4. Place the chopped leeks in a large bowl full of water and swish vigorously. Make several water changes, rinsing the leeks until free of sand. Drain well.

Chopping and Cleaning Kale, Collards, and Other Hearty Greens

1. Holding the greens in a bunch, trim off the bottom inch or so of the stems.

2. Still holding them in a bunch, thinly slice the remaining stems.

3. When you reach the leaves, roll the stack into a fat cigar shape and continue slicing as thin as possible.

4. Give the cutting board a quarter-turn and thinly slice the leaves in the opposite direction. Rinse thoroughly in a bowl full of water, and change the water repeatedly until free of sand. Drain well.

Quick Tip: Some recipes may advise you to trim off and discard the stems and thick midribs of hearty greens, but this is somewhat wasteful and not usually necessary.

Stemming and Washing Spinach

Young, tender spinach does not need stemming, but the thick, fibrous stems of older leaves should be discarded.

1. Fold each leaf in half in one hand, grab the stem end with the other, and pull gently; discard the stem and toss the leaves in a large bowl full of water as you go.

2. Swish vigorously. Lift from the water, empty, and rinse bowl. Repeat the process until the spinach is free of sand.

Quick Tip: Triple-washed packaged spinach is a handy alternative to washing spinach yourself.

Dicing Green and Red Bell Peppers

1. Cut in half lengthwise and remove the stem, seeds, and any thick white membranes.

2. Set shiny side down and cut thin strips lengthwise.

3. Line up the strips and cut crosswise.

Shredding Cabbage

1. Discard any bruised or limp outer leaves.

2. Quarter the cabbage and slice away the hard central core.

3. Slice each quarter as thinly as possible or pass through the feed tube of a food processor fitted with a shredding disk.

Mincing Fresh Ginger

1. Remove the peel with a paring knife.

2. Slice as thinly as possible lengthwise.

3. Pile up the slices and again cut thinly lengthwise.

4. Give the stack a quarter-turn, then slice crosswise.

Quick Tip: If you are using a food processor, toss small pieces of ginger through the feed tube into the empty bowl while the motor is running.

BASIC POTS AND PANS

Having a great set of knives will only get you halfway through your food preparations. You also need the right pots and pans. Your first selection should be a good-quality 12-inch nonstick skillet with a lid, a pan you'll use repeatedly in the Soy Zone kitchen. It can even double as a wok for stir-frying vegetables, tempeh, and tofu. Look for one that has a heavy bottom with an aluminum or copper sandwich for even heating. Buy the best you can afford; All-Clad is an excellent choice.

For making soups and stews, you'll need a heavy ovenproof 6-quart saucepan with a lid, sometimes known as a Dutch oven. Le Creuset makes a line of enameled cast-iron models that are expensive but superb.

A pressure cooker will be essential if you are cooking frequently with dried beans. This will dramatically reduce both time and effort, two important requirements in the Soy Zone kitchen.

The final tools you'll need are two types of measuring cups. For dry ingredients, get nesting measuring cups that come in 1-cup, $1/2$-cup, $1/3$-cup, and $1/4$-cup sizes. Purchase Pyrex glass liquid measuring cups in the quart and 2-cup sizes. For best results, avoid using a liquid measuring cup for dry ingredients and vice versa. It's handy to have two or three sets of measuring spoons so you don't have to keep rinsing and drying as you go.

Miscellaneous Kitchen Tools

Here are some other useful (not to mention fun) kitchen tools you may want to acquire:

Bowls—light, nesting stainless steel bowls ranging from large to small

Box grater—for grating carrots and citrus

Electric mini-chopper—a quick way to mince garlic and ginger

Immersion blender—an inexpensive electric appliance that makes quick work of pureeing soups right in the pot. Some models come with canister attachments for making smoothies and chopping garlic and ginger. Braun is a good brand.

Pepper mill—for optimum flavor, freshly ground pepper is highly recommended. The Purex brand imported from France is preferred by many chefs.

Salad spinner—indispensable for quickly drying masses of greens in a jiffy. Zyliss makes a good one.

Steaming basket—an inexpensive aluminum basket on short legs that allows food to sit above the water while cooking

Vegetable peeler—Good Grips makes two excellent models

Kitchen scissors—a surprisingly useful tool for opening plastic packages and snipping fresh herbs

Long-handled rubber spatulas and wooden spoons—for mixing and stirring

Spring-loaded tongs—great for turning things over, including peppers roasting over the burner

Understanding Common Cooking Terms

Once you have all the recipe ingredients ready to go, you must cook them properly. As with food preparation, there are numerous cooking terms that you need to know in order to understand recipes.

Boiling: Cooking food in a liquid, usually water. You'll know that food has come to a boil when there are lots of bubbles on the surface.

Blanching: Quickly cooking a vegetable in a large quantity of boiling water just long enough (usually only a minute or two) to tenderize slightly, leach out bitterness, or facilitate removal of skin (like tomatoes).

Braising: Slow-cooking in a covered pot using a small quantity of liquid.

Broiling: Cooking food directly under the heat source.

Frying: Cooking uncovered over high heat in oil or in a nonstick pan.

Grilling: Cooking food directly above the heat source, either wood or charcoal, which imparts a pleasantly smoky flavor.

Roasting/Baking: Cooking food in a preheated oven.

Simmering: Cooking at a gentle boil.

Steaming: Cooking food in a tightly covered pot over boiling liquid.

Stir-frying: As the name implies, frying with rapid stirring so that the contact between the pan and food ingredients is of a relatively short duration.

You've got your kitchen stocked with you favorite Soy Zone foods. You've got all the latest kitchen gadgets. Now it's time to sink your teeth into some great-tasting, easy recipes. The next chapter should be an adventure. *Zone appétit!*

Soy Zone Meals

Getting into the Soy Zone involves more than supplementing your meals with soy products. You need to get a balance of protein, carbohydrate, and fat in order to reap the full health benefits that soy has to offer. In other words, you *must* eat meals that will keep your insulin levels in the Zone—not too high and not too low. Just as importantly, your Soy Zone meals must be easy to prepare, pleasing to the eye, and taste even better than the same-old meals that you make every night.

To meet these formidable challenges, I called on a consortium of vegetarian chefs to formulate meals that are incredibly easy to incorporate into your daily dietary lifestyle. Each is balanced in terms of protein, carbohydrate, and fat so that all you have to do is follow the recipe and enjoy. What's more, you'll get 25 to 30 grams of protein in each serving, so you don't have to worry about whether you're getting too little protein or too much.

This chapter includes more than 100 breakfast, lunch, snack, and dinner recipes. All of these meals will take you into the Zone, and virtually all contain a healthy dose of soy protein. Many of the recipes contain no animal protein, so they are suitable for vegans and non-vegetarians alike. These recipes are marked with a "vegan" symbol.

I've also included recipes that combine soy protein with other low-fat protein sources such as chicken, fish, and low-fat dairy products. These combination recipes will show you how easy it is to fit soy into your meal plan. In other words, if you're not a vegan, you don't need to become one in order to follow the Soy Zone.

Trying out a new recipe is like taking yourself on a little adventure. You never know quite what to expect when preparing the meal, nor how your family will react when you serve it. (Truth is, you're not taking a big risk. You can always try out a recipe once and decide it's not for you.) Take this opportunity to revel in your new cooking experiences. Remember, variety is the spice of life, and I think I've included enough variety to please even the pickiest of palates. You're bound to find at least three or four meals that will become new family favorites. Also note that each recipe contains the number of Zone Food Blocks for each ingredient. These Zone Food Blocks, which are explained in greater detail in Chapter 7, allow you to make ingredient changes without affecting the hormonal response to the meal.

Think of these meals as a gift you're giving to yourself and your loved ones. You're giving the gift of good home-cooked food, but, more importantly, you're giving the gift of good health.

A SAMPLE WEEKLY MENU

Monday
Breakfast: Banana-Berry Sundae
Lunch: Tofu Enchiladas
Snack 1: Zone Strawberry Ice Cream
Dinner: Baked Golden Dumplings with Saucy Dip
Snack 2: Cinnamon Peaches with Ricotta

Tuesday
Breakfast: Spinach and Tofu Quicherole
Lunch: Tofu Vegetable Kebabs
Snack 1: Zoned Muffins
Dinner: Chunky Miso Soup
Snack 2: Very Berry Smoothie

Wednesday
Breakfast: Cheese and Veggie Melt
Lunch: Tureen of Curried Tempeh, Tofu, and Vegetables

Snack 1: Zone Cocoa-Banana Freeze
Dinner: Stir-Fry Tofu with Peppers and Peanuts
Snack 2: Apple Kanten with Maple Tofu

Thursday
Breakfast: Asparagus Frittata
Lunch: Tomato Fennel Soup with Tofu Basil Pistou
Snack 1: Blueberry Muffin
Dinner: Easy Bar-B-Q Tempeh and Vegetables
Snack 2: Nectarine Freeze

Friday
Breakfast: Cheddar-Apple "Galette"
Lunch: Three Bean Salad with Smoked Tofu and Mustard
Snack 1: Peaches-n-Cream Yogurt Smoothie
Dinner: Tempeh Taco Salad
Snack 2: Chocolate Yogurt with Fruit

Saturday
Breakfast: Mediterranean Gratin
Lunch: Cold Tempeh Salad
Snack 1: Zoned Muffins
Dinner: Individual Baked Tofu Soufflés with Gravy and Roasted
    Vegetables
Snack 2: Lemon Meringue

Sunday
Breakfast: Sicilian Cauliflower Egg Frittata with Sausage and
    Peppers
Lunch: Vietnamese Spring Lettuce Rolls with Peanut Dressing
Snack 1: Classic Antipasto
Dinner: Barley Mushroom Soup
Snack 2: Peaches and Cream Yogurt Smoothie

THE SOY ZONE
Breakfast Dishes

Sicilian Cauliflower and Egg Frittata with Sausage and Peppers

Servings: 1 Breakfast Entrée (4 blocks)

Block size	Ingredients
1/2 carbohydrate	2 cups cauliflower florets
1 protein	1 whole egg
1 1/2 protein	3 egg whites
4 fat	1 1/3 teaspoons olive oil
1 carbohydrate, 1 1/2 protein	1 1/2 links "Lite Life" Italian tofu sausage
1/2 carbohydrate	1 small onion, sliced
1/2 carbohydrate	1 large green pepper, sliced
1/2 carbohydrate	1 ripe tomato, sliced into wedges
1 carbohydrate	1 cup strawberries, sliced

Instructions

1. Cut off thick stem of cauliflower and discard. Separate cauliflower into florets by hand or with a knife. Chop remaining stalk or discard.

2. Rinse and steam cauliflower in steamer basket over boiling water, or in small amount of water with no basket, until tender, about 10 minutes. Drain and mash gently with fork.

3. Beat egg and egg whites together. Put 2/3 teaspoon olive oil in a frying pan (non-stick, preferably) and heat on low. Add cauliflower evenly in pan and cook until lightly browned. Add eggs and cover. Keep flame as low as possible and cook frittata until almost done on top.

4. Loosen frittata around edges. Place serving dish large enough to cover frying pan over top. Flip frittata onto dish and immediately slip back into frying pan. Cook 3 to 5 minutes longer until browned on second side. Set aside.

5. Break up sausage into bite-size pieces. Put $^1/_3$ teaspoon olive oil in pan (cast iron, preferably) and spread with pastry brush. Add sausage and sauté on medium-high heat, stirring frequently until brown. Remove from pan.

6. Add remaining $^1/_3$ teaspoon olive oil to same pan and sauté onion 3 to 5 minutes with 2 tablespoons water. Add green pepper and sauté 2 to 3 minutes, then add fresh tomato. There should be a little gravy. If not, add more water or broth, then cover and heat through for up to 5 minutes over low heat.

7. Serve frittata with sausage and pepper and onion mixture on the side.

8. Serve strawberries on the side.

Apple and Cheese Melt

Servings: 1 Breakfast Entrée (4 blocks)

Block size	Ingredients
	$^1/_4$ to $^1/_3$ cup purified water (less for a gas range; more for electric)
	$^1/_4$ teaspoon powdered cinnamon or ginger
1 carbohydrate	1 tablespoon raisins
3 carbohydrate	1 to 1$^1/_2$ small (5 to 6 oz) apples, halved and cut into eighths or 2-inch cubes (Jonathan, Jonagold, Braeburn, Rome, Fuji, or Granny Smith)
4 protein	4 ounces low-fat mozzarella or cheddar-style soy cheese, grated or cut in thin strips
4 fat	12 almonds, raw or lightly toasted

Instructions

1. Add water, spice, and raisins to an 8- or 9-inch skillet with a lid. If cooking for two, use two small skillets or one 10- or 12-inch skillet; for four people, use a 12- to 13-inch skillet.

2. Wash apples; peel if desired. Halve apples and scoop out inner core with a teaspoon, grapefruit spoon, or melon baller. Slice and add to skillet. Cover and bring to boil. Reduce heat and simmer for about 4 to 6 minutes, until almost tender.

3. Meanwhile, weigh cheese unless it comes in 1-ounce logs (as is the case with string cheese) and grate. Remove lid from skillet; sprinkle nuts, then cheese over fruit. Cover and simmer for 2 to 3 minutes until cheese melts, then remove from heat. Or simply sprinkle on cheese, cover, and remove from heat.

4. Use a spatula to slide apple and cheese onto a dinner plate. Serve immediately.

Cherry-Berry Yogurt Smoothie

Servings: 1 Breakfast Entrée (4 blocks)

Block size	Ingredients
2 protein, 2 carbohydrate	1 cup plain low-fat yogurt (increase to 1⅓ cups if using yogurt made without non-fat dry milk added)
2 protein	⅔ ounce unflavored or unsweetened vanilla soy protein powder (portion containing 14 grams protein)
	½ teaspoon pure vanilla extract (non-alcohol, glycerine base)
	⅛ teaspoon ground nutmeg or powdered ginger
	⅛ to ¼ teaspoon stevia extract powder
1 carbohydrate	½ cup frozen, unsweetened blueberries

1 carbohydrate	3/4 cup frozen, unsweetened cherries
4 fat	1 1/3 teaspoons almond oil
	or 2 teaspoons almond or cashew butter
	Optional: 3 to 4 ice cubes

Instructions

1. Place yogurt and protein powder in the blender. Cover and bend until smooth; top and scrape down the sides with a spatula if needed. Add flavorings, spices, frozen fruit, and oil or nut butter. Blend until smooth. Taste. For added thickness, add 3 to 4 ice cubes, then blend until thick, creamy, and icy.

2. Serve immediately or refrigerate in a small jar or chilled thermos bottle, then serve within 24 hours.

Variations

Cherry-Cantaloupe Yogurt Smoothie: Replace 1/2 cup blueberries with 3/4 cup cantaloupe. Prepare as above.

Cherry-Berry Kefir Smoothie: Replace yogurt about with 1 cup plain, unsweetened kefir, then add an extra 1/3 ounce protein powder (portion containing 7 grams protein). Prepare as above.

Banana-Berry Sundae

Servings: 1 Breakfast Entrée (4 blocks)

Block size	Ingredients
4 fat	12 almonds
4 protein	1 cup low-fat cottage cheese
	1/2 to 1 teaspoon pure vanilla extract
	1/8 teaspoon ground cinnamon
1 carbohydrate	1/3 large banana, cut in slices lengthwise
3 carbohydrate	1 1/2 cups fresh or frozen berries, thawed

Instructions

1. Preheat oven to 350°F.

2. On baking sheet, spread almonds. Toast in oven until golden brown and almonds give off aroma, about 7 to 10 minutes. Watch carefully so they don't burn. Set aside.

3. In medium bowl, combine cottage cheese, vanilla extract, and cinnamon.

4. Arrange banana slices around the outer rim of a serving bowl. With ice cream scoop, shape cottage cheese mixture into mounds in serving bowl. Top with berries. Sprinkle with nuts.

Variations

Replace banana with 1 cup sliced fresh strawberries.

If using non-fat cottage cheese, double amount of almonds. (When using zero-fat protein foods, you need to add an extra fat block for each protein block.)

Overnight Maple Nut Oatmeal

Servings: 1 Breakfast Entrée (4 blocks)

Block size	Ingredients
4 carbohydrate	$2/3$ cup non-instant *rolled* oats
	$1/8$ teaspoon sun-dried sea salt
	$1\frac{1}{3}$ cups boiling purified water
4 protein	$1\frac{1}{3}$ ounce unflavored or unsweetened vanilla soy protein powder (portion containing 28 grams protein)
	$1/8$ to $1/4$ teaspoon apple pie spice
	1 teaspoon pure maple extract (in a non-alcohol, glycerine base)
	$1/4$ teaspoon white stevia extract powder **or** 4 drops stevia extract liquid

4 fat   12 almonds **or** 4 macadamia nuts, raw or
                                                         lightly toasted, chopped coarsely

Instructions (for thermos oats)

1. Add rolled oats and sea salt to a wide-mouth (preferably stainless steel) thermos bottle. Add boiling water. Immediately cover tightly with a lid. Allow to sit out on the counter overnight.

2. In the morning, stir thoroughly with a wide wooden spoon. Transfer to a large cereal bowl. Add protein powder, spice, flavoring extract, and stevia. Stir well to dissolve lumps. Top with chopped nuts. Serve immediately or quickly transfer to thermos bottle; cover, then take to work for breakfast.

Instructions (for Crock-Pot)

1. Just before going to bed, add rolled or steel-cut oats and sea salt to a mini-Crock-Pot (called a Crockette; do not use a large Crock-Pot for a small volume of cereal; unit must be filled at least half-full or too much water will evaporate). Add *cold* water. Set dial to the lowest setting.

2. Cover and allow to cook all night. In the morning, turn off heat. Let stand for 10 to 15 minutes. Stir thoroughly with a wooden spoon. Transfer to a large cereal bowl. Add protein powder, spice, flavoring extract, and stevia. Stir well to dissolve lumps. If soy protein is used, you may need to add additional hot water, a few tablespoons at a time, to create a smooth mixture. Top with chopped nuts. Serve immediately or quickly transfer to thermos bottle; cover, then take to work for breakfast.

Mediterranean Gratin

Servings: 1 Breakfast or Dinner Entrée (4 blocks)

Block size	Ingredients
	3 to 4 tablespoons purified water
	1 clove garlic, minced
	1/2 teaspoon dried oregano
	1/8 teaspoon ground black pepper
1/2 carbohydrate	1 small yellow onion, chopped
1/4 carbohydrate	1/2 medium red bell pepper, seeded, diced
1/4 carbohydrate	1/2 medium yellow bell pepper, seeded, diced
1/3 carbohydrate	1 1/3 cups cremini or button mushrooms, thinly sliced
1/3 carbohydrate	1 1/3 cups broccoli florets and stems, peeled and finely chopped
1/3 carbohydrate	1 1/3 cups cauliflower florets
1 carbohydrate	1 medium carrot, peeled, thinly sliced
4 fat	12 olives, pitted, sliced
	Scant bread crumbs
4 protein	4 ounces soy cheese, grated
1 carbohydrate	1/2 cup grapes

Instructions

1. Preheat oven to 400°F.

2. In sauté pan that has a cover and can go into the oven, put water, garlic, oregano, and pepper. Stir in onion, red and yellow pepper, mushrooms, broccoli, cauliflower florets, and carrot. Bring to boil over high heat, then reduce to low heat and simmer, covered, for about 6 to 10 minutes, or until vegetables are tender. (Add water if needed.)

3. Remove lid from skillet and add olives. Sprinkle scant bread crumbs and grated cheese onto vegetables. Place skillet, uncovered, in oven and bake until cheese melts, about 4 to 6 minutes. Use spatula to transfer vegetable melt to serving plate. Garnish with grapes and eat for dessert.

Cheddar-Apple "Galette"

Servings: 1 Breakfast Entrée (4 blocks)

Block size	Ingredients
	¼ to ⅓ cup purified water
	¼ teaspoon ground cinnamon
1 carbohydrate	1 tablespoon raisins
3 carbohydrate	1½ small apples, such as Granny Smith or Fuji, halved, cored, and cut into eighths
4 fat	4 walnut halves, chopped
4 protein	4 ounces sharp low-fat cheddar cheese, grated

Instructions

1. Preheat oven to 400°F.

2. In medium sauté pan that has a lid and can go into the oven, add water, cinnamon, raisins, and apples. Bring to boil over high heat, then reduce to medium, cover, and simmer until apples are tender, about 6 to 10 minutes.

3. Uncover pan and turn off heat. With a wooden spoon or spatula, group apple slices together to form a loose circle. Sprinkle with chopped walnuts and grated cheese. Transfer pan to oven and cook until cheese melts, about 3 to 5 minutes. Serve hot.

Asparagus Frittata

Servings: 1 Breakfast or Dinner Entrée (4 blocks)

Block size	Ingredients
2 protein	4 ounces extra-firm tofu, cubed
1 protein	1 whole egg **or** 2 egg whites
1 protein	2 egg whites
	1/4 teaspoon ground turmeric
	1/8 to 1/4 teaspoon ground black pepper
	1/4 teaspoon sun dried sea salt **or** 1 teaspoon tamari soy sauce
1 carbohydrate	1/2 cup unsweetened tomato sauce
1/2 carbohydrate	1/2 cup onion, cut in rings
2 carbohydrate	2 cups asparagus, chopped
1/2 carbohydrate	1 cup yellow bell pepper strips
4 fat	1 1/3 teaspoons olive oil

Instructions

1. Mash tofu in a medium bowl. Add egg, whites, spices, and sea salt or tamari. Whisk with a fork. Set aside. Gently warm tomato sauce in a small saucepan over low heat.

2. Layer vegetables on a metal steamer basket, and set in a 1 1/2-quart pot filled with 1/2 inch purified water. Cover and bring to boil. Reduce heat to medium and steam for 5 to 6 minutes or until just tender. Immediately transfer vegetables from pot to a serving plate with a large slotted spoon.

3. Heat oil in a 9-inch skillet. (Use a larger skillet for two people.) Heat over medium-high flame until oil sizzles. (Pan must be hot or eggs will stick!) Tilt skillet to coat evenly.

4. Pour in egg mixture all at once, then reduce heat to medium-low. As eggs begin to set up (almost immediately), push cooked portion aside with a spatula, then let uncooked portion run under. Repeat as eggs start to set up. Keep moving spatula.

Cook for about 3 to 4 minutes or until eggs are cooked throughout but still glossy and moist.

5. Remove from heat before eggs become dry. Transfer to serving plate. Top vegetables or eggs with tomato sauce.

Variation

Reduce tofu in the recipe above to 2 ounces. When scramble is done cooking, sprinkle on 1 ounce of shredded, part-skim mozzarella cheese.

Very Berry Smoothie

Servings: 1 Breakfast Entrée (4 blocks)

Block size	Ingredients
1 carbohydrate	1/3 cup unsweetened pineapple juice
4 protein	Unflavored soy protein powder (portion containing 28 grams protein)
	1/2 teaspoon pure vanilla extract (non-alcohol, glycerin base)
	1/8 teaspoon ground nutmeg
2 carbohydrate	1 cup frozen, unsweetened blueberries
1 carbohydrate	1 heaping cup frozen, unsweetened strawberries
4 fat	1 1/3 teaspoons peanut oil

Instructions

1. Place juice and protein powder in blender container. Cover and blend until smooth.

2. Add vanilla, nutmeg, blueberries, strawberries, and peanut oil. Blend until smooth, scraping down sides of blender if necessary.

Variations

For sweeter smoothie, add ⅛ teaspoon stevia extract powder. For added thickness or iciness, add 4 to 6 ice cubes. Blend until smooth.

Vegan Strawberry-Cantaloupe Smoothie: Replace blueberries with 1½ cups frozen, cubed cantaloupe. Blend until smooth.

Vegan Strawberry-Peach Smoothie: Replace blueberries with 1½ cups frozen, cut peaches (from 2 peaches). Blend until smooth.

Zoned Cocoa-Banana Cherry Freeze

Servings: 1 Breakfast Entrée (4 blocks)

Block size	Ingredients
¾ protein, ¾ carbohydrate	½ cup Edensoy Original Soy Milk or similar brand, chilled
4 fat	4 teaspoons unsweetened almond or macadamia nut butter (see Note below)
3¼ protein	1 ounce + 1 tablespoon unflavored or unsweetened vanilla soy protein powder (portion containing 23 grams protein)
¼ carbohydrate	1 heaping tablespoon unsweetened cocoa powder
	1 teaspoon pure vanilla extract (non-alcohol, glycerine base)
	Optional: ⅛ to ¼ teaspoon stevia extract powder or 2 to 4 drops stevia extract liquid
	Optional: 1 tablespoon apple fiber powder
1 carbohydrate	⅓ ripe, medium banana, peeled, sliced, and frozen (about ⅓ cup)

2 carbohydrate

1½ cups frozen, unsweetened cherries

Optional: 3 to 4 ice cubes (from purified water)

Instructions

1. Pour soy milk into a blender container. Add nut butter, protein powder, unsweetened cocoa, vanilla, and stevia. Add apple fiber powder if desired (for added thickness and blood sugar control). Cover and blend until smooth. Stop and scrape down the sides with a spatula.

2. With motor running, add frozen fruit through the top feeder. When blended, add ice cubes one or two at a time, blending on the ice-crushing setting until desired thickness. Stop and start blender, pushing the pulse button repeatedly until ice is completely crushed and mixture is smooth and thick. Try a spoonful. Add more stevia if a sweeter taste is desired.

3. Pour into four custard cups or dessert dishes and serve immediately, or 4 to 8 small paper cups, then freeze until firm, about 3 hours. If frozen solid, remove from freezer 10 to 15 minutes before serving, or as needed to soften to an ice cream texture. Alternatively, pour into a tall fountain glass to serve one person for breakfast.

Note: Normally 2 teaspoons of nut butter would count as four fat blocks; however, protein powders contain no added fat, so the amount of fat used in this recipe was doubled in order to create a Zoned ratio. If nut butter had not been increased, recipe would be too low in fat and less satisfying or sustaining.

Zoned Blueberry Muffins

Servings: 1 Breakfast Entrée (4 blocks) or 4 Snacks (1 block each)

Block size	Ingredients
	Non-stick spray
	Oat flour to dust pans (prevent sticking)
2 carbohydrate	1/3 cup oat flour
3 protein	1 ounce unflavored protein powder (whey protein, egg white protein, or soy protein—see Note; 21 grams protein)
	3/4 teaspoon non-aluminum baking powder
	1/4 teaspoon ground ginger
	1/4 teaspoon ground cinnamon
	1 pinch ground nutmeg
	1/8 teaspoon finely ground sea salt
	3/4 teaspoon stevia extract powder
1 carbohydrate	1/3 cup unsweetened apple juice
1 protein	1 whole egg
4 fat	2 2/3 teaspoons almond or sesame oil
	1 teaspoon pure vanilla extract (non-alcohol, glycerine base)
1 carbohydrate	1/2 cup fresh blueberries or 2/3 cup frozen, unsweetened blueberries

Instructions

1. Preheat oven to 375°F.

2. Liberally oil 4 muffin tins (do not oil the remaining muffin tins). Dust tins with oat flour to prevent sticking.

3. In a 1 1/2-quart mixing bowl, sift oat flour and protein powder. Add baking powder, ginger, cinnamon, nutmeg, salt, and stevia. Sift and set aside.

4. In a small bowl combine apple juice, egg, oil, and vanilla. Whisk with a fork. Add to dry ingredients and stir until evenly mixed and no lumps remain.

5. Using half the batter, fill each prepared muffin tin about half-way. Evenly distribute blueberries among cups. Top with remaining batter.

6. Bake for 20 to 30 minutes or until firm to the touch and lightly golden around the edges. A toothpick inserted in the middle should come out clean. Allow to cool at least 10 minutes. Run a knife around the sides of muffins to release from the pan. Cool. Refrigerate and use within one week or freeze.

Notes: If protein powder is from soy protein, add an additional 1/4 cup water to batter.

Muffins will be fluffier and rise better with egg white or whey protein powder.

Overnight Egg Nog Oatmeal

Servings: 1 Breakfast Entrée (4 blocks)

Block size	Ingredients
4 carbohydrate	2/3 cup rolled oats
	1/8 teaspoon sun-dried sea salt
	1 1/3 cup boiling purified water
4 protein	1 1/3 ounce unsweetened protein powder
	1/8 to 1/4 teaspoon ground nutmeg
	1 teaspoon pure vanilla extract (non-alcohol, glycerin base)
	1/4 teaspoon white stevia extract powder **or** 4 drops stevia extract liquid
4 fat	1 1/3 teaspoon almond or walnut oil (or 12 almonds or 4 macadamia nuts, raw or lightly toasted, chopped coarsely)

Instructions

1. Add rolled oats and sea salt to a wide-mouth thermos bottle. Add boiling water. Immediately cover tightly with a lid. Allow to sit overnight.

2. In the morning, stir thoroughly with a wide wooden spoon and transfer to a large cereal bowl. Add protein powder, nutmeg, vanilla, and stevia. Stir well to dissolve lumps. Top with oil or chopped nuts. Serve immediately or return to thermos bottle to serve later.

Variation (Crock-Pot cooking)

1. Just before bedtime, add rolled or steel-cut oats and sea salt to a mini-Crock-Pot. (Do NOT use a large Crock-Pot for a small volume of cereal. Unit must be at least half-full or too much water will evaporate during cooking.) Add cold water. Set dial to the lowest setting.

2. Cover and cook all night. In the morning, turn off heat. Let stand for 10 to 15 minutes. Stir thoroughly with a wooden spoon. Transfer to a large cereal bowl.

3. Add protein powder, nutmeg, vanilla, and stevia. Stir well to dissolve lumps. If soy protein is used, you may need to add additional hot water, a few tablespoons at a time, to create a smooth mixture. Top with oil or chopped nuts. Serve immediately or transfer to thermos bottle to serve later.

Pear and Cheese Melt

Servings: 1 Breakfast Entrée (4 blocks)

Block size	Ingredients
	¼ to ⅓ cup purified water (less for a gas range; more for electric)
	¼ teaspoon powdered anise or whole anise seeds
1 carbohydrate	1 tablespoon raisins or currants **or** 2 dates, minced
3 carbohydrate	1½ small or 1 medium pear (7 ½ ounces total), Anjou, Comice, Bartlett, or Bosc pears, halved, cored, and cut into thin wedges

| 4 protein | 4 ounces low-fat mozzarella, Colby, Monterey Jack, or cheddar-style soy cheese, grated or cut in thin strips |
| 4 fat | 12 lightly toasted almonds, or 4 macadamia nuts, coarsely chopped |

Instructions

1. Add water, spice, and raisins to an 8- or 9-inch skillet with a lid. If cooking for two, use two small skillets or one 10- to 12-inch skillet.

2. Wash pears; peel if waxed. Halve pear and scoop out inner core with a teaspoon or melon baller. Slice and add to skillet. Cover and bring to boil. Reduce heat and simmer for about 4 to 6 minutes, or until almost tender. While fruit cooks, grate cheese.

3. Remove lid from skillet; sprinkle nuts, then cheese over fruit. Cover and simmer for 2 to 3 minutes or until cheese melts. Or simply sprinkle over fruit, cover, remove from heat, and let stand 3 to 4 minutes until cheese melts.

4. Remove from heat. Use a spatula to slide pear and cheese onto a dinner plate. Serve immediately.

Variations

Replace the 12 almonds or 4 macadamia nuts with 12 toasted pecan halves. Prepare as above.

Peachy Cheese Melt: Replace $1^1/_2$ small pears with $1^1/_2$ peaches. Use anise seed or powder or replace with cinnamon.

Scrambled Eggs with "Sausage" and Veggies

Servings: 1 Breakfast Entrée (4 blocks)

Block size	Ingredients
1 protein	1 whole egg
1 protein	2 egg whites
	1/4 teaspoon turmeric powder
	1/8 teaspoon mild red pepper powder (Ancho, Anaheim, or Chipotle)
	1/2 teaspoon rice vinegar or raw apple cider vinegar
	1/2 teaspoon tamari soy sauce
	Optional: 1 to 2 tablespoons minced scallions
2 fat	2/3 teaspoon olive oil
2 protein, 1 1/2 carbohydrate, 2 fat	3 Light Life Lean Links, cut into thin slices or diced
	1/4 inch purified water (to barely cover bottom of skillet or sauté pan)
	1 teaspoon tamari soy sauce
	1/4 teaspoon ground black pepper or dry mustard
1/2 carbohydrate	1/2 cup onion, cut into half-moon slices
1 carbohydrate	1 (16-ounce) package frozen, chopped spinach
1 carbohydrate	1/2 apple, sliced

Instructions

1. Whisk eggs, turmeric, red pepper, vinegar, and tamari. Add scallions if desired. Set aside.

2. Heat a wok, cast-iron skillet, or 9- to 10-inch skillet over medium heat. Add oil and tilt to coat. When hot, add egg mixture. As soon as the bottom of the eggs start to

firm, toss in "sausage." Scramble with a fork or metal spatula, lifting up cooked portion and allowing uncooked portion to run underneath. Cook until eggs are barely firm. Immediately remove from heat and transfer to a 10-inch serving plate.

3. For spinach: Add water to a 9- to 10-inch skillet, then tamari or sea salt, spice, onion, then frozen spinach. Cover and bring to a boil. Reduce heat and simmer for 4 to 6 minutes or until spinach is tender. Remove lid during the last few minutes to cook away excess liquid.

4. Transfer spinach to the plate with the eggs. Serve with apple on the side.

Variation

Replace 3 Lean Links with some other brand of vegetarian sausage with a similar profile. If the sausage you select is higher in carbohydrates, simply reduce the amount of spinach eaten, saving the rest for another meal.

Spinach and Tofu Quicherole with Fruit Salad

Servings: 1 Breakfast or Dinner Entrée (4 blocks)

Block size	Ingredients
1/2 carbohydrate	8 ounces (half a 16-ounce package) frozen spinach, thawed
	1/2 teaspoon finely ground sea salt
1 protein	2 ounces extra-firm or 3 ounces firm tofu, mashed
1 protein	2 egg whites
2 protein	2 ounces low-fat Monterey Jack cheese or part-skim mozzarella, grated
4 fat	2 teaspoons roasted sesame tahini
1/2 carbohydrate	1 tablespoon dried onion flakes
	1 teaspoon tamari
	1/2 clove garlic, minced or pressed
	1/2 teaspoon dry mustard (powder)

¼ teaspoon ground black pepper

Optional: 1 teaspoon nutritional yeast flakes

Accompaniments:

1 carbohydrate	½ cup grapes or blueberries
1 carbohydrate	1 cup fresh or thawed, unsweetened strawberries or raspberries
1 carbohydrate	1 peach or plum, halved, pitted, and sliced
	2 teaspoons fresh lemon, lime, or orange juice
	½ teaspoon vanilla extract (non-alcohol, glycerine base)
	⅛ teaspoon ground nutmeg
	4 macadamia nuts or 12 almonds or pecans, lightly toasted, chopped

Instructions

1. Preheat oven to 350°F. Oil one shallow 6-ounce ramekin dish. Set aside.

2. Place thawed spinach in a large mixing bowl. Sprinkle with sea salt, mix with your hands for several minutes, until spinach wilts and releases moisture. Let stand for 10 to 15 minutes. Meanwhile, combine tofu, egg, cheese, tahini, dried onion, tamari, and spices in a 2-quart mixing bowl. Mix with a large wooden spoon.

3. Pick up one handful of spinach. Squeeze out as much water as you can, then transfer the wilted spinach to the mixing bowl with tofu. Repeat with remaining spinach. Discard spinach water. Mix tofu-spinach combination to evenly distribute seasonings. Transfer to prepared baking pan. Smooth the top with a wooden spoon or spatula.

4. Bake in preheated oven for 20 minutes or until firm to the touch and lightly golden around the edges. While casserole bakes, wash and slice fruit. Combine in a 16- to 24-ounce bowl. Mix citrus juice, vanilla, and spice in small dish. Stir, then pour over fruit. Add nuts. Toss gently.

5. Allow to cool for 10 minutes. Alternatively, cover and chill, then serve cold with fruit salad.

Variations

Reduce cheese to 1 ounce, then increase tofu to 4 ounces firm or extra-firm tofu.

Prepare a double batch to serve two people, or prepare a quadruple batch in a 10-inch pie plate, to serve four people or two meals for two. If using a pie plate, bake for 40 to 50 minutes.

Acerola Cherry Yogurt

Servings: 1 Breakfast Entrée (4 blocks) or 4 Snack Portions (1 block each)

Block size	Ingredients
4 carbohydrate	2 cups plain low-fat yogurt
4 protein	14 grams soy protein powder
	1/2 teaspoon pure vanilla extract (non-alcohol, glycerine base)
	1 rounded teaspoon acerola cherry powder (from the health food store)
	1/8 teaspoon ground nutmeg or powdered ginger
	1/4 teaspoon stevia extract powder
4 fat	1 1/3 teaspoons almond oil, or 12 almonds, raw or lightly toasted, chopped coarsely

Instructions

1. Place yogurt in small bowl or 1-quart Pyrex measuring cup. Add soy protein powder, vanilla, acerola powder, nutmeg or ginger, and half of the stevia powder. Stir well with a large spoon, scraping the sides as needed to incorporate all of the seasonings.

2. Taste. Add the rest of the stevia if a sweeter taste is desired. Stir in almond oil or sprinkle nuts on top.

3. Serve now or pour into one container for breakfast or four containers for snacks. Cover and refrigerate.

Variation

Egg Nog–Flavored Kefir: Replace yogurt with plain, unflavored kefir (goat's milk yogurt, available at natural foods stores).

Breakfast Sundae

Servings: 1 Breakfast Entrée (4 blocks)

Block size	Ingredients
4 protein	1 cup low-fat cottage cheese
	3/4 teaspoon pure vanilla or maple extract (non-alcohol, glycerine base)
	1/8 teaspoon ground nutmeg or cinnamon
1 carbohydrate	1/3 large banana, cut in half lengthwise
1 carbohydrate	1/2 cup blueberries, fresh or frozen and thawed
1 carbohydrate	1 fresh peach, pitted and sliced
1 carbohydrate	8 cherries, pitted, fresh or frozen and thawed
4 fat	12 almonds, toasted lightly, chopped coarsely, or 12 walnut or pecan halves, chopped coarsely

Instructions

1. Combine cottage cheese, vanilla or maple extract, and spice in a medium-sized bowl.

2. Arrange banana halves around the outer rim of a large cereal bowl or dinner plate. Use an ice cream scoop to shape cottage cheese and arrange on top of or in between banana halves.

3. Top with blueberries, sliced peach, then cherries. Sprinkle nuts on top.

Serving suggestions: Serve immediately.

Variations

Replace banana with 1 cup sliced, fresh strawberries, arranged in a circle around the outside of the serving bowl.

If using non-fat cottage cheese, double the amount of nuts used. The reason: when using zero-fat protein foods, you need to add an extra fat block for each protein block.

Fruit Salad with Almond Cream

Servings: 1 Breakfast Entrée (4 blocks) or 4 Snack or Dessert Portions (1 block each)

Block size	Ingredients
1 carbohydrate	1 cup "original" flavored almond milk (Pacific Foods of Oregon is a well-known brand)
	2 tablespoons agar flakes (vegan equivalent of gelatin, found in natural foods stores)
4 protein	$1\frac{1}{3}$ ounces unflavored protein powder (portion containing 28 grams soy protein)
4 fat	4 teaspoons unsweetened almond, hazelnut, or pistachio butter
	1 tablespoon pure vanilla or maple extract (non-alcohol, glycerine base)
	$\frac{1}{2}$ teaspoon stevia extract powder
	$\frac{1}{4}$ cup purified water
1 carbohydrate	$\frac{3}{4}$ cup frozen cherries, thawed before use
1 carbohydrate	1 peach, halved, pitted, sliced
1 carbohydrate	$\frac{1}{3}$ medium banana, sliced, or $\frac{1}{2}$ cup blueberries

Instructions

1. Pour almond milk into a 1-quart saucepan and sprinkle agar flakes on top. Bring to boil over medium heat. Reduce heat and simmer for 5 minutes until agar is dissolved and mixture is smooth. Stir periodically with a wooden spoon.

2. Pour almond milk mixture into a blender. Cover and blend for 30 seconds. Add protein powder, nut butter, vanilla, and stevia powder. Blend until smooth. Scrape down the sides of the blender with a spatula as needed to incorporate the powder.

3. Pour mixture into 12-ounce bowl. Chill for 2 to 3 hours or until firm to the touch.

4. Cut mixture into pieces with a large spoon and put back in the blender. Blend until smooth and creamy. Add water only as needed to blend. Chill again.

5. Combine fresh fruits in a large serving bowl and top with nut cream. For dessert, divide fruit between 4 soup bowls or wine goblets and top with nut cream.

Variations

Replace $3/4$ cup cherries with $3/4$ cup diced cantaloupe.

Replace peach with 2 kiwis, peeled and sliced in thin rounds.

Replace banana or blueberries with $1/2$ cup seedless grapes.

Picnic-Style Cold Tempeh Salad with "Mayo"

Servings: 1 Lunch Entrée (4 blocks)

Block size	Ingredients
2 protein, 2 carbohydrate	4 ounces tempeh, cubed into 1/4-inch pieces
	1 tablespoon tamari sauce
3 fat	1 1/2 tablespoons Nayonaise (tofu mayonnaise)
1/2 carbohydrate, 1/2 protein	1/4 cup plain yogurt
1/2 carbohydrate	Juice of 1/2 lemon
	2 teaspoons prepared mustard
1/2 carbohydrate	3 medium celery stalks, chopped
1/2 carbohydrate	1 medium green pepper, diced
1 1/2 protein	3 hard-boiled egg whites, chopped
	1 slice of red onion, diced
1 fat	3 black olives, sliced
	1 medium sprig fresh dill or parsley, minced

Instructions

1. Preheat oven to 350°F.

2. Toss tempeh with tamari sauce in baking dish and bake uncovered for 10 to 12 minutes. Set aside to cool.

3. Mix Nayonaise, yogurt, lemon juice, and mustard. Add celery, green pepper, egg whites, and red onion.

4. Fold in tempeh cubes and sprinkle with olives and herbs.

5. Chill and serve on a bed of lettuce, if desired.

Tofu "Cottage" and Green Salad

Servings: 1 Lunch Entrée (4 blocks)

Block size	Ingredients
4 protein	12 ounces firm tofu, mashed with a fork 1 teaspoon ume vinegar/umeboshi vinegar (not the same as regular vinegar) **or** 1 teaspoon dulse granules (flaked, purple sea vegetable, rich in minerals, sold in natural foods stores)
3 fat	1 tablespoon light mayonnaise **or** 3 tablespoons Nayonaise (tofu mayonnaise)
1/4 carbohydrate	1/2 cup celery, finely minced
1/4 carbohydrate	1/3 packed cup sweet onion (Walla Walla or Vidalia), finely minced
1/4 carbohydrate	1/2 cup minced red/yellow bell pepper or combination
1 carbohydrate	4 teaspoons pickle relish (preferably unsweetened)
1 carbohydrate	1/3 cup water chestnuts, chopped coarsely 1 tablespoon dried **or** 3 tablespoons fresh, minced chives
1/4 carbohydrate	2 1/2 cups red leaf or green leaf lettuce, shredded
1/4 carbohydrate	1/2 cup cucumber, peeled, cut in thin slices
1/2 carbohydrate	1 cup cherry tomatoes

| 1 fat | 3 olives, chopped coarsely |
| | **or** 3 almonds or walnut halves or pecan halves, raw or lightly toasted, chopped |

Instructions

1. Combine tofu, umeboshi vinegar or dulse, mayonnaise, celery, onion, bell pepper, pickle relish, water chestnuts, and chives in a medium-sized bowl. Stir to evenly distribute.

2. Arrange lettuce on a serving plate. Top with cucumber. Arrange tomatoes in a circle around the outside edges of the plate. Pack tofu mixture into a small bowl and invert over lettuce. Top with chopped olives or nuts. Serve immediately or cover and refrigerate until later.

Variation

Cottage Cheese and Green Salad: Omit tofu, umeboshi/dulse, and mayonnaise. Replace with 1 cup low-fat cottage cheese. Mix with chopped vegetables, pickle relish, 2 teaspoons lemon juice, water chestnuts, and chives. Serve over raw veggies, topped with 12 olives or 12 lightly toasted, chopped almonds or walnuts. If using non-fat cottage cheese, double the amount of nuts or olives used in order to create a Zone balance.

Salad Nicosia

Servings: 1 Lunch Entrée (4 blocks)

Block size	Ingredients
1½ carbohydrates	2 small new potatoes
½ carbohydrate	1 small head red leaf or green leaf lettuce, washed, patted dry, and shredded
½ carbohydrate	½ medium cucumber, peeled, quartered, thinly sliced
½ carbohydrate	1 tomato, cut into wedges

¼ carbohydrate	½ yellow bell pepper, seeded, diced
¼ carbohydrate	½ small sweet onion (Walla Walla or Vidalia), sliced into thin rings
1 protein	1 ounce non-fat Swiss or cheddar cheese, cut into thin strips
2 protein, ½ carbohydrate	4 slices Fat-Free Yves Veggie Deli slices
1 protein	1 hard-boiled egg, quartered
4 fat	2 tablespoons Nayonaise (tofu mayonnaise)
	1 to 2 tablespoons purified water
	1 teaspoon prepared mustard
	1 teaspoon red wine vinegar
	Pinch of salt, or to taste
	⅛ teaspoon black pepper
	¼ teaspoon dried basil

Instructions

1. Scrub potatoes with cold water and cut into ¼-inch slices. Put into small saucepan and cover, with an extra inch, of water. Bring to boil. Turn heat down to medium, to a slight rolling boil, and cook potatoes until they feel tender when poked with a fork, about 10 to 12 minutes. Drain and cool.

2. Arrange lettuce leaves on serving plate. Top with cucumber, tomato, yellow pepper, and onion. Layer on sliced potatoes, then cheese. Roll up individual "deli" slices and arrange over cheese. Arrange egg wedges around salad.

4. In a small bowl, combine Nayonaise, water (add more or less for desired consistency), mustard, vinegar, salt, pepper, and basil. Pour over salad. Serve.

Note: Salad can be made ahead and refrigerated in container with airtight lid. Keep dressing to the side until ready to serve.

Variation

Omit cheese and egg, and replace with 3 to 4 ounces smoked tofu, cut into thin strips.

Oriental Chef's Salad

Servings: 1 Lunch Entrée (4 blocks)

Block size	Ingredients
1/4 carbohydrate	2 1/2 cups prewashed Spring Salad Mix or Mesclun Greens or romaine lettuce, shredded or torn
3/4 carbohydrate	1/2 medium cucumber, peeled, halved, thinly sliced
1 1/2 carbohydrate	1/2 cup water chestnuts, sliced
1/2 carbohydrate	1 cup *each* broccoli and cauliflower, cut in florets
1/4 carbohydrate	1 cup red radishes, cut into thin slices
	1/4 cup scallions, thinly sliced on the diagonal
1/4 carbohydrate	1/2 yellow or orange bell pepper, seeded, cut into long thin strips
4 protein, 1/2 carbohydrate	4 to 6 ounces firm, seasoned tofu, such as smoked tofu, cubed or cut into julienne strips
	Optional: 1 teaspoon dulse granules (purple sea vegetable, rich in minerals, found in natural foods stores)
4 fat	2 tablespoons Nayonaise (tofu mayonnaise)
	1 tablespoon purified water
	1 teaspoon prepared mustard
	1 teaspoon tamari soy sauce
	1/8 teaspoon ground black pepper or red pepper
	Optional: 1/8 teaspoon dried basil, oregano, or dill weed, crumbled

Instructions

1. Arrange salad greens, cucumber, and water chestnuts on a serving plate or in a portable bowl with a snap-on lid.

2. Layer and spread vegetables out in the order listed on a collapsible vegetable steamer or bamboo steamer basket over rapidly boiling water. Cover and steam for 6 to 8 minutes or until crisp-tender. Immediately transfer basket of vegetables to the sink. Run cold (preferably purified) water over them to stop the cooking and hold their brilliant colors. Drain thoroughly.

3. Arrange cooked, cooled vegetables over salad greens in concentric circles around the plate or in sections: one pile of broccoli next to a pile of cauliflower, next to red radishes, then scallions, and bell pepper strips. Arrange sliced seasoned tofu in the center of the plate or fanned out across the vegetables.

4. Combine Nayonaise, water, mustard, and tamari. Stir, then pour over salad. Season with pepper and basil. Serve immediately or cover and refrigerate until later.

Variation

For convenience, wash and chop two or three times as many vegetables as you need. Store each kind in a separate pint or quart jar in the refrigerator for easy access and quick salad fixing over the next few days. They won't get lost because you will see them at a glance when you open the fridge. Their vibrant colors will entice you to eat them! Works every time!

Vietnamese Spring Lettuce Rolls with Peanut Dressing

Servings: 1 Lunch Entrée (4 blocks)

Block size	Ingredients
4 protein	8 ounces extra-firm tofu, cubed
1 carbohydrate	½ cup carrots, grated
⅓ carbohydrate	1 cup bean sprouts, washed and dried

1/3 carbohydrate	2 stalks bok choy, washed and shredded
1/4 carbohydrate	1/2 small sweet onion, such as Walla Walla or Vidalia, grated
1/2 carbohydrate	1/2 cucumber, peeled and grated
1/4 carbohydrate	1/2 red bell pepper, cut in 1/4-inch strips
1/4 carbohydrate	1/2 yellow bell pepper, cut in 1/4-inch strips
	1 tablespoon fresh mint, finely chopped
3 fat	1 tablespoon peanut oil
	2 teaspoons lime juice
	1 teaspoon rice wine vinegar
	1 to 2 inches gingerroot, peeled and grated to equal 2 teaspoons
	1 tablespoon chives, chopped
	1/4 teaspoon salt, or to taste
1/2 carbohydrate	6 large red leaf or green leaf lettuce leaves, washed and patted dry
1 fat	6 peanuts, finely chopped

Instructions

1. In a medium bowl, combine tofu, carrots, bean sprouts, bok choy, onion, cucumber, red and yellow pepper, and fresh mint. Set aside.

2. In a jar with lid, put peanut oil, lime juice, rice wine vinegar, ginger, chives, and salt. Close lid and shake dressing until well mixed. Taste and adjust seasoning.

3. Coat tofu and vegetables with dressing and toss together. Spoon equal amounts of mixture onto lettuce leaves, sprinkle peanuts, and roll up. Serve chilled.

Smoked Tofu and Green Salad

Servings: 1 Lunch Entrée (4 blocks)

Block size	Ingredients
4 fat	2 teaspoons sesame tahini
	2 tablespoons hot purified water
	1 teaspoon red wine vinegar or apple cider vinegar
	1 teaspoon tamari soy sauce
	1/2 teaspoon wet mustard (Dijon or stone ground)
	1/8 teaspoon ground black pepper or mild red pepper
1/2 carbohydrate	2 1/3 cup Spring Salad Mix, Mesclun Mix, or dark leaf lettuce, shredded or torn into small pieces
3/4 carbohydrate	1/2 medium cucumber, peeled, halved, thinly sliced
1/4 carbohydrate	1/2 red or yellow bell pepper, halved, seeded, diced
1/2 carbohydrate	1 cup cherry tomatoes or low-acid gold pear tomatoes
1 carbohydrate	1/3 small sweet potato, baked, peeled, sliced thinly
1/4 carbohydrate	1/2 cup celery, cut into long, thin diagonal slices
1/4 carbohydrate	1 cup red radishes, cut into thin slices
4 protein, 1/2 carbohydrate	4 1/2 to 6 ounces smoked or firm seasoned tofu, cubed

Instructions

1. Combine dressing ingredients in a small mortar and pestle. Mix until smooth and creamy. Pour into a small custard cup, cover, and refrigerate for several hours or overnight to thicken.

2. Layer salad ingredients in the order listed on 1 large dinner plate or in a portable 1-quart bowl with a snap-on lid. Top with cubed, smoked tofu. Cover and refrigerate.

3. Just before serving, add dressing to salad, stir, then serve.

Notes: For convenience make a double, triple, or quadruple batch of dressing, then portion into small jars or custard cups with snap-on lids and refrigerate for use over the course of several days or the week.

You can also wash and chop two or three times as many vegetables as you need. Store each kind in a separate pint or quart jar in the refrigerator for easy access and quick salad fixing over the next few days. They won't get lost because you will see them at a glance when you open the fridge. Their vibrant colors will entice you to eat them! Works every time!

Teriyaki Tofu Salad

Servings: 1 Lunch Entrée (4 blocks)

Block size	Ingredients
4 protein	8 ounces plain, extra-firm tofu, cubed
1 carbohydrate	1 tablespoon teriyaki sauce
	3 tablespoons vegetable broth or purified water
4 fat	1⅓ teaspoons sesame oil, raw or toasted variety
1 carbohydrate	4 cups broccoli, cut into florets, stems peeled and sliced into thin rounds (or use half broccoli, half cauliflower)
¼ carbohydrate	¾ cup scallions, white and green part, cut into 1-inch logs
¼ carbohydrate	½ cup celery, cut into thin diagonal slices
¼ carbohydrate	1 cup red radishes or Japanese white radish, cut into thin slices
¼ carbohydrate	½ red or orange bell pepper, halved, seeded, diced
1 carbohydrate	1 cup carrot, cut julienne or thin half-moons

Instructions

1. Arrange cubed tofu in a 12- to 16-ounce bowl. Combine teriyaki sauce, broth, and sesame oil. Pour over tofu, gently stir to coat. Cover and refrigerate for at least 3 hours or overnight, turning once or twice to season all sides.

2. Layer and spread vegetables on a collapsible vegetable steamer or bamboo steamer basket over rapidly boiling water, in the order listed. Cover and steam for 6 to 8 minutes or until crisp-tender. Immediately transfer basket of vegetables to the sink. Run cold (preferably purified) water over them to stop the cooking and hold their brilliant colors. Drain thoroughly.

3. Arrange vegetables on a large dinner plate or in a portable 1-quart bowl with a snap-on lid. Top with cubed, seasoned tofu and any remaining marinade. Serve now or cover and refrigerate.

Variation

Use 4 to 5 ounces of commercial Teriyaki tofu in the recipe above, then omit teriyaki sauce, broth, oil, and marinating step. Read labels for fat content; brands vary considerably.

Note: Chop up two, three, or four times as many vegetables as you need for this dish, then store each kind in a separate glass jar in the refrigerator. You'll have the makings of quick-steamed, stir-fried, or sautéed vegetable dishes. Use the vegetables within three to five days.

Tofu Antipasto

Servings: 1 Lunch Entrée (4 blocks)

Block size	Ingredients
1/4 carbohydrate	2 1/2 cups red leaf or green leaf lettuce, shredded
3/4 carbohydrate	1/2 medium cucumber, peeled, quartered, cut in thin slices
1/2 carbohydrate	1 tomato, cut into wedges **or** 1 cup cherry tomatoes
1/4 carbohydrate	1/2 yellow bell pepper, seeded, cubed or diced
1/4 carbohydrate	1/4 cup sweet white onion (Vidalia or Walla Walla Sweets), cut into rings or half-moons **or** frozen, thawed pearl onions
1 1/2 carbohydrate	1/4 cup + 2 tablespoons chickpeas, cooked, drained
1 protein	1 ounce low-fat Swiss or cheddar cheese–style soy cheese, julienne cut, diced or grated
2 protein	4 slices Fat-Free Yves Veggie Deli slices **or**
1/2 carbohydrate	3 slices Fat-Free Yves Canadian Veggie Bacon, sliced or diced
1 protein	1 hard-boiled egg or two hard-boiled whites, peeled, cut into wedges
	Optional: 1 teaspoon dulse granules (a purple sea vegetable, rich in minerals with a salty flavor, sold in natural foods stores)
4 fat	4 tablespoons Nayonaise (tofu mayonnaise)

1 to 2 tablespoons purified water

1 teaspoon prepared mustard

1 teaspoon tamari soy sauce

1/8 teaspoon ground black pepper or red
     pepper

Optional: 1/4 teaspoon dried basil, oregano, or
     dill weed, crumbled between your fingers

Instructions

1. Arrange lettuce on a serving plate or in a portable bowl with a snap on lid. Top with remaining vegetables, then cheese, sliced "deli meats," and egg, arranged in concentric circles around the plate or in sections. Sprinkle with dulse granules if desired.

2. Combine Nayonaise, water, mustard, tamari, and spice in a small dish. Stir, then pour over salad. Serve immediately or cover and refrigerate until later.

Notes: For convenience, wash and chop two or three times as many vegetables as you need. Store each kind in a separate pint or quart jar in the refrigerator for easy access and quick salad fixing over the next few days. They won't get lost because you will see them at a glance when you open the fridge. Their vibrant colors will entice you to eat them! Works every time!

Because zero-fat protein foods were used for all or most of the protein blocks in this recipe, the amount of tofu mayonnaise was increased to give you a 40–30–30 ratio.

Variation

Omit soy cheese and egg; replace with 3 to 4 ounces smoked tofu, cut into thin strips or cubes.

Peaches-n-Cream Yogurt Smoothie

Servings: 4 Snack Portions (1 block each) or 1 Breakfast Entrée (4 blocks)

Block size	Ingredients
2 protein, 2 carbohydrate	1 cup plain low-fat yogurt (increase to 1$\frac{1}{3}$ cups if using yogurt made without non-fat dry milk added)
2 protein	$\frac{2}{3}$ ounce unflavored protein powder, preferably unsweetened egg white or whey protein powder.
	$\frac{1}{2}$ teaspoon pure vanilla extract, (non-alcohol, glycerine base)
	$\frac{1}{8}$ teaspoon ground nutmeg or powdered ginger
	$\frac{1}{8}$ teaspoon stevia extract powder
2 carbohydrate	2 whole peaches, cut up and frozen
4 fat	1$\frac{1}{3}$ teaspoons almond oil, or 2 teaspoons unsweetened almond or cashew butter
	Optional: 3 to 4 ice cubes

Instructions

1. Place yogurt and protein powder in the blender. Cover and blend until smooth. Stop blender and scrape down the sides with a spatula, if needed.

2. Add vanilla, nutmeg or ginger, stevia, frozen peaches, and oil or nut butter. Blend until smooth. For added thickness, add 3 to 4 ice cubes, then blend until thick, creamy, and icy.

Serving suggestions: Serve immediately or refrigerate in a small jar or chilled thermos bottle. Serve within 24 hours.

Variations

Peaches-n-Cream Kefir Smoothie: Replace yogurt about with 1 cup plain, unsweetened kefir, then add an extra $1/3$ ounce protein powder. Prepare as above.

Nectarine-n-Cream Smoothie: Replace peaches above with 1 whole nectarine, halved, pitted, sliced, preferably frozen. Prepare as above.

Chocolate Yogurt with Fruit

Servings: 4 Snack Portions (1 block each)

Block size	Ingredients
2 protein, 2 carbohydrate	1 cup plain low-fat yogurt
2 carbohydrate	2 cups fresh strawberries, sliced, or 1 cup strawberries and $1/3$ banana, sliced
	$2^{1/2}$ teaspoons unsweetened cocoa powder
2 protein	$2/3$ ounce unflavored soy protein powder (portion containing 14 grams protein)
	2 teaspoons apple fiber powder (found in natural foods stores, it adds thickness and fiber)
	$3/4$ teaspoon pure vanilla extract (non-alcohol, glycerine base)
	$1/4$ teaspoon stevia extract powder
4 fat	$1^{1/3}$ teaspoons almond oil, or 12 almonds, raw or lightly toasted, chopped coarsely
	Ground nutmeg, to garnish

Instructions

1. Combine yogurt and fruit in a blender. Cover and blend until smooth. Add cocoa powder, protein powder, apple fiber powder, vanilla, and half the stevia powder. Blend, scrape down sides as needed to incorporate powder, and blend again until smooth.

2. Taste, and add the rest of the stevia if a sweeter taste is desired. Stir in almond oil or sprinkle nuts on top. Dust with ground nutmeg.

3. Pour into one container for breakfast or four containers for snacks. Cover and refrigerate for at least 3 hours to allow flavors to mingle and mixture to thicken. Top with sliced fruit before serving.

Variations

Replace fruit with 2 blocks' worth of your favorite fruit. Try cherries, blueberries, apricots, peaches, mango, and ripe pears.

Chocolate Yogurt with Cherries on Top: Allow $1^1/_2$ cups frozen, unsweetened cherries to thaw for at least 4 to 6 hours in a bowl in the refrigerator. Spoon over chocolate yogurt just before serving.

Blueberry Yogurt

Servings: 4 Snack Portions (1 block each) or 1 Breakfast Entrée (4 blocks)

Block size	Ingredients
2 protein, 2 carbohydrate	1 cup plain low-fat yogurt
2 carbohydrate	1 cup fresh or frozen, unsweetened blueberries
2 protein	$^2/_3$ ounce unflavored soy protein powder (portion containing 14 grams protein)
	2 teaspoons apple fiber powder (found in natural foods stores, it adds thickness and fiber)
	$^3/_4$ teaspoon pure vanilla extract (non-alcohol, glycerine base)
	$^1/_4$ teaspoon stevia extract powder
4 fat	$1^1/_3$ teaspoons almond oil or 12 almonds, raw or lightly toasted, chopped coarsely
	Ground nutmeg, to garnish

Instructions

1. Combine yogurt and fruit in a blender. Cover and blend until smooth. Add protein powder, apple fiber powder, vanilla, and half the stevia powder. Blend, scrape down sides as needed to incorporate powder, and blend again until smooth.

2. Taste, and add the rest of the stevia if a sweeter taste is desired. Stir in almond oil or sprinkle nuts on top. Dust with ground nutmeg.

3. Pour into one container for breakfast or four containers for snacks. Cover and refrigerate for at least 3 hours to allow flavors to mingle and mixture to thicken. Top with sliced fruit before serving.

Variations

Replace blueberries with 2 blocks' worth of your favorite fruit. Try cherries, apricots, peaches, and ripe pears.

"Egg Nog" Yogurt with Fruit

Servings: 4 Snack Portions (1 block each) or 1 Breakfast Entrée (4 blocks)

Block size	Ingredients
2 protein, 2 carbohydrate	1 cup plain low-fat yogurt
2 protein	2/3 ounce unflavored or unsweetened vanilla soy protein powder (portion containing 14 grams protein)
	1/2 to 1 teaspoon pure vanilla extract (non-alcohol, glycerine base)
	Scant 1/8 teaspoon turmeric powder
	1/8 teaspoon ground nutmeg
	1/8 to 1/4 teaspoon stevia extract powder (start with less; add more only if needed)
4 fat	1 1/3 teaspoons almond oil **or** 12 almonds, raw or lightly toasted, chopped coarsely
1 carbohydrate	1/3 banana, cut in thin slices
1 carbohydrate	1 peach, halved, pitted, sliced

Instructions

1. Place yogurt in small bowl or 1-quart Pyrex measuring cup. Add protein powder, vanilla, turmeric, nutmeg, and stevia. Stir well with a large spoon, scraping the sides as needed to incorporate all of the seasonings. Taste. Add $1/8$ teaspoon additional stevia if a sweeter taste is desired. Stir in almond oil or sprinkle nuts on top.

2. Top with sliced fruit just before serving. Serve immediately or pour into one container (for a breakfast) or four containers (to yield four snacks). Cover and refrigerate.

Note: If slicing fruit in advance of serving, either drizzle it with lemon juice or place it in the bottom of serving containers, then top with "Egg Nog" Yogurt.

Variations

Replace banana with 2 dates, chopped finely.

Replace 1 peach with $1/2$ cup blueberries. If desired, also replace $1/3$ banana with $1/2$ cup blueberries. (You do not need to coat blueberries with lemon juice, only sliced fruit, sliced in advanced of serving.)

Vegan Berry Smoothie

Servings: 4 Snack Portions (1 block each) or 1 Breakfast Entrée (4 blocks)

Block size	Ingredients
1 carbohydrate	$1/3$ cup unsweetened apple or pineapple juice
4 protein	$1 1/2$ ounces unflavored soy protein powder (portion containing 28 grams protein)
	$1/2$ teaspoon pure vanilla extract (non-alcohol, glycerine base)
	$1/8$ teaspoon ground nutmeg or powdered ginger

2 carbohydrate	1 cup blueberries, frozen and unsweetened
1 carbohydrate	1 heaping cup strawberries, frozen and unsweetened
4 fat	1$\frac{1}{3}$ teaspoons almond oil, or 2 teaspoons almond or cashew butter
	Optional: $\frac{1}{8}$ teaspoon stevia extract powder
	Optional: 4 to 6 ice cubes

Instructions

1. Place juice and protein powder in the blender. Cover and blend until smooth. Scrape down the sides with a spatula if needed. Add vanilla extract, spice, frozen fruit, and oil or nut butter. Blend until smooth.

2. Taste. Add stevia if additional sweetness is desired. For added thickness, add 4 to 6 ice cubes two at a time, with the motor running. Blend until thick, creamy, and icy.

Serving suggestions: Serve immediately or refrigerate in a small jar or chilled thermos bottle. Serve within 24 hours.

Variations

Vegan Strawberry-Cantaloupe Smoothie: Replace each 1 cup blueberries with 1$\frac{1}{2}$ cups frozen, cubed cantaloupe.

Vegan Strawberry-Peach Smoothie: Replace each 1 cup blueberries with 1$\frac{1}{2}$ cups frozen, cut-up peaches (about 2 whole peaches).

Peach-Protein Popsicles

Servings: 4 Snack or Dessert Portions (1 block each)

Block size	Ingredients
2 carbohydrate	2/3 cup unsweetened apple, pear, or pineapple juice
4 fat	2 teaspoons unsweetened almond, hazelnut, or pistachio butter
4 protein	1 1/3 ounces unflavored soy protein powder (portion containing 28 grams protein)
	2 teaspoons pure vanilla extract (non-alcohol, glycerine base)
2 carbohydrate	2 peaches, halved, pitted, sliced
	Optional: 1/4 teaspoon stevia extract powder

Instructions

1. Combine juice, nut butter, protein powder, and vanilla in the blender. Blend. Scrape down the sides with a spatula as needed to mix in powder and dissolve lumps. Blend again until smooth. Add fruit, and blend. Taste, then add stevia powder if a sweeter taste is desired.

2. Pour into eight Popsicle molds. Affix the plastic tops with the built-in stick and holder. Freeze at least 3 to 4 hours, until firm.

3. To serve, run warm water over the outside of each mold to loosen pops and allow for easy removal.

Notes: If you don't have plastic Popsicle molds, simply use small paper cups. Arrange the cups on a small cake pan, fill, and freeze 1 to 2 hours. When the mixture starts to ice up, insert a Popsicle stick into the center of each cup. Freeze until firm.

Or, forget the Popsicle idea altogether! Pour the mixture into four 8-ounce paper cups, freeze, and eat with a spoon.

Variations

Raspberry-Peach Protein Popsicles: Replace 1 peach with 1 cup fresh or frozen raspberries.

Strawberry-Peach Protein Popsicles: Replace 1 peach with 1 cup strawberries. Use sesame tahini or sunflower butter in place of the nut butter.

Melon-Cherry Protein Pops

Servings: 4 Snack or Dessert Portions (1 block each)

Block size	Ingredients
	1/3 cup purified water, plus slightly more as needed to blend
4 fat	2 teaspoons unsweetened almond or hazelnut butter, or 1 1/3 teaspoons almond or hazelnut oil
	1/4 teaspoon stevia extract powder
2 carbohydrate	1 1/3 cups honeydew melon, in chunks
4 protein	1 1/3 ounces unflavored protein powder (portion containing 28 grams protein)
	2 teaspoons pure vanilla or maple extract (non-alcohol, glycerine base)
2 carbohydrate	3/4 cups frozen, unsweetened, pitted cherries

Instructions

1. Combine water, nut butter or oil, stevia powder, and melon in the blender and blend until smooth. Add protein powder and flavoring extract and blend until smooth. Scrape down the sides with a spatula as needed to mix in powder and dissolve lumps. Add cherries and blend, adding a little more water as needed to create a smooth texture.

2. Pour into eight Popsicle molds. Affix the plastic tops with the built-in stick and holder. Freeze at least 3 to 4 hours, until firm.

3. To serve, run warm water over the outside of each mold to loosen pops and allow for easy removal.

Notes: If you don't have plastic Popsicle molds, simply use small paper cups. Arrange the cups on a small cake pan, fill, and freeze 1 to 2 hours. When the mixture starts to ice up, insert a Popsicle stick into the center of each cup. Freeze until firm.

Or, forget the Popsicle idea altogether! Pour the mixture into four 8-ounce paper cups, freeze, and eat with a spoon.

Variations

Blueberry-Honeydew Protein Pops: Replace $^3/_4$ cup cherries with 1 cup fresh blueberries.

Cherry-Cantaloupe Pops: Replace $1^1/_3$ cups honeydew melon with $1^1/_2$ cups cantaloupe.

Lunch or Dinner Entrées

Tofu Enchiladas

Servings: 1 Lunch or Dinner Entrée (4 blocks)

Block size	Ingredients
Filling	
2 protein	4 ounces extra-firm tofu
	1 tablespoon shoyu sauce
	1 cup spinach, washed and chopped
2 fat	$2/3$ teaspoon olive oil
	1 tablespoon chili powder, or to taste
	Onion powder, to taste
	Garlic powder, to taste
$1/4$ carbohydrate	2 tablespoons tomato puree
2 protein	4 ounces low-fat ricotta cheese
Sauce	
$1/4$ carbohydrate	$1/2$ small onion, sliced
$1/2$ carbohydrate	1 medium green pepper, sliced
2 fat	$2/3$ teaspoon olive oil
1 carbohydrate	$1/2$ cup tomato puree
	1 tablespoon chili powder
	1 teaspoon garlic powder
	Salt and pepper, to taste
	$1/4$ cup water
2 carbohydrate	Two 6-inch corn tortillas

Instructions

1. Freeze tofu, defrost, squeeze dry, and tear into bite-size pieces. Toss with shoyu sauce.

2. Cook spinach in a small pot with ¼ cup water 3 to 5 minutes. Remove from heat and set aside.

3. Sauté tofu in oil with chili powder, onion powder, garlic powder, and seasoning for 3 minutes. Add the 2 tablespoons tomato puree, stir, and remove from heat. Mix with ricotta and spinach and set aside.

4. Preheat oven to 350°F.

5. Sauté onion and peppers in oil. Add the ½ cup tomato puree and seasoning. Cook 15 to 20 minutes. Add water after 10 minutes to make a thin sauce.

6. Dip each tortilla in warm sauce to make it soft and easy to work with. Fill with tofu and fold both sides in.

7. Pour ⅓ of sauce in a baking pan. Lay enchiladas on top and cover with remaining sauce. Bake at 350°F for 20 minutes covered, then 5 minutes uncovered. Serve on a bed of raw spinach, if desired.

Tofu-Vegetable Kebabs with Yogurt Olive Dip

Servings: 1 Lunch or Dinner Entrée (4 blocks)

Block size	Ingredients
Dip	
½ protein, ½ carbohydrate	¼ cup plain low-fat yogurt
1 fat	3 black olives, sliced
	2 teaspoons prepared mustard
½ carbohydrate	1 teaspoon honey
	Optional: ½ teaspoon light miso
	1 medium sprig fresh parsley, minced
Kebabs	
1 carbohydrate	2 medium zucchini, cubed
½ carbohydrate	1 large onion, cut into small chunks

3½ protein	7 ounces extra-firm tofu, cubed
1 carbohydrate	12 mushrooms, whole
3 fat	1 teaspoon olive oil
	Salt and pepper, to taste
½ carbohydrate	6 whole cherry tomatoes

Instructions

1. Mix yogurt, olives, mustard, honey, miso, and parsley. Set aside.

2. Blanch zucchini and onion in boiling water for two minutes and drain. Onion may separate, which is to be expected.

3. Alternate tofu, zucchini, onion, and mushroom on skewers, always ending with mushroom. Brush with olive oil, and lightly salt and pepper. Put under broiler or on outdoor grill. Turn after 5 minutes and grill another 5 minutes.

4. Serve with yogurt-olive dip and cherry tomatoes.

Tomato Fennel Soup with Tofu and Basil Pistou

Servings: 1 Lunch or Dinner Entrée (4 blocks)

Block size	Ingredients
Soup	
2 carbohydrate	3 medium fresh tomatoes, diced (4 if canned)
½ carbohydrate	1 small fennel bulb, sliced thin
1 carbohydrate	2 medium onions, diced
	1 clove garlic, minced
	2 cups water
	2 tablespoons vegetable broth powder
4 protein	8 ounces extra-firm tofu, cubed

Pistou

	3 to 4 whole stalks fresh basil (parsley, if basil is out of season)
3 fat	1 teaspoon olive oil
½ carbohydrate	Juice of ½ lemon
	Dash salt
	½ teaspoon light miso, yellow or white
1 fat	3 black olives, sliced

Instructions

1. Combine tomatoes, fennel, onion, garlic, water, vegetable broth powder, and tofu in large soup pot. Heat to boiling and then simmer on low, covered, for 30 minutes.

2. Meanwhile, combine basil, olive oil, lemon juice, salt, miso, and olives in small food processor (also use small blender, mortar and pestle, or suribachi) and grind to coarse paste.

3. Serve soup in bowls and add dollop of basil pistou to taste in the center. Stir pistou in while eating.

Variation

Put tofu on lightly oiled cookie sheet and cover with Italian seasoning. Bake for 10 to 15 minutes at 350°F. Serve with pistou.

Tureen of Curried Tempeh, Tofu, and Vegetables

Servings: 1 Lunch or Dinner Entrée (4 blocks)

Block size	Ingredients
Curry	
4 fat	1⅓ teaspoons peanut oil
	2 tablespoons curry spice, or to taste
	2 cups vegetable broth
½ carbohydrate	¼ cup tomato puree
	Optional: ½ teaspoon saffron
	1 clove garlic, pressed
	1 teaspoon fresh ginger, grated
½ carbohydrate	1 small onion, chopped
½ carbohydrate	6 green beans
	6 wax beans
¼ carbohydrate	1⅓ cups cauliflower, cut into small pieces
1½ protein, 1½ carbohydrate	3 ounces extra-firm tofu
1½ protein	3 ounces tempeh
Raita	
1 protein, 1 carbohydrate	½ cup plain yogurt
	¼ teaspoon sugar
	Dash salt
	Dash cayenne pepper
	½ clove garlic, pressed
	1 small sprig parsley, minced
	Optional: 1 sprig fresh cilantro, minced

Instructions

1. Heat oil on low in large frying pan or sauté pan and whisk in curry. Roast curry for 10 to 12 seconds to enhance flavor, being careful not to burn. Add broth, tomato puree, saffron, garlic, and ginger. Bring to boil.

2. Add onion, beans, cauliflower, tofu, and tempeh and lower heat. Simmer covered for 15 to 20 minutes, or to desired tenderness. Add water or vegetable broth to make more soupy.

3. Mix yogurt, sugar, salt, pepper, garlic, parsley, and cilantro. Serve as a cooling sauce over curry.

Stuffed Zucchini

Servings: 1 Lunch or Dinner Entrée (4 blocks)

Block size	Ingredients
1 carbohydrate	2 medium zucchini
2 protein	4 ounces extra-firm tofu
	1 tablespoon shoyu sauce
	Garlic powder, to taste
2 fat	$2/3$ teaspoon olive oil
1 protein	2 ounces low-fat ricotta cheese
2 fat	$2/3$ teaspoon olive oil
1/2 carbohydrate	1 small onion, chopped
1/4 carbohydrate	2 medium stalks celery, chopped
1/4 carbohydrate	6 mushrooms, chopped
1 carbohydrate	$2^{1}/2$ tablespoons dry oatmeal
1 protein	1 egg, beaten
1 carbohydrate	1/2 cup tomato sauce
	Fresh seasonal herbs, minced

Instructions

1. Preheat over to 350°F.

2. Leave zucchini ends intact and blanch or steam for 5 to 7 minutes. Cut in half lengthwise. Remove pulp but leave enough meat so the zucchini will stand upright.

3. Mash tofu with a fork and integrate shoyu sauce. Add garlic powder and sauté in olive oil in a skillet for 2 to 3 minutes. Remove from heat and add to ricotta in separate bowl.

4. Add olive oil to same skillet and sauté onion, celery, and mushroom until slightly browned. Add to tofu-ricotta mixture with oatmeal and egg.

5. Stuff zucchini boats and place in baking dish on a layer of tomato sauce. Top with remaining tomato sauce and herbs. Bake 20 minutes, covered, at 350°F. Uncover and bake 5 minutes longer.

Zone-Friendly Vegetarian Pad Thai

Servings: 1 Lunch or Dinner Entrée (4 blocks)

Block size	Ingredients
Sauce	
	2 tablespoons apple cider vinegar
	2 to 3 tablespoons tamari or shoyu sauce
1 carbohydrate	2 teaspoons brown sugar
2 fat	1 teaspoon natural peanut butter
Sauté	
2 fat	$2/3$ teaspoon peanut oil
1 protein	1 egg, beaten
3 protein	6 ounces extra-firm tofu, cubed
	2 cloves garlic, minced
	2 scallions, chopped, white and green parts separated

	1 teaspoon hot pepper, minced or dash
	Optional: Crushed red pepper
1 carbohydrate	2 cups mung bean sprouts
	4 to 5 water chestnuts
1 carbohydrate	1 lime in wedges
1 carbohydrate	Tossed salad, large, containing two sliced tomatoes
	Tamari sauce
	$\frac{1}{2}$ clove garlic, minced

Instructions

1. Combine vinegar, tamari, brown sugar, and peanut butter and stir until smooth. Set aside.

2. Add $\frac{1}{3}$ teaspoon oil to skillet and cook beaten egg until firm. Remove and set aside.

3. Put remaining oil in same skillet and sauté tofu, garlic, white part of scallions, and crushed red pepper for 2 to 3 minutes. Add bean sprouts and heat on high until wilted, about 3 to 4 minutes, stirring frequently. Add water chestnuts and mix together gently.

4. Stir in peanut butter sauce and heat over low flame until warm. Top with green part of scallions and a lime wedge and serve with tossed salad dressed with lime juice, dash of tamari, and garlic.

Variation

Egg may be omitted. Cube 8 ounces of tofu instead of 6 ounces.

Three-Bean Salad with Smoked Tofu and Mustard Vinaigrette

Servings: 1 Lunch or Dinner Entrée (4 blocks)

Block size	Ingredients
1 carbohydrate	1½ cups green beans or yellow wax beans, or combination, trimmed, washed, and cut in half on the diagonal
½ carbohydrate	1 small onion, thinly sliced
	2 teaspoons umeboshi vinegar
	1 tablespoon brown rice vinegar or red wine vinegar
4 fat	1⅓ teaspoons olive oil
	2 teaspoons prepared mustard, such as Dijon
	2 tablespoons parsley, minced
	1 clove garlic, minced
1 carbohydrate	¼ cup canned garbanzo beans, drained and rinsed
1 carbohydrate	¼ cup canned kidney beans, drained and rinsed
4 protein, ½ carbohydrate	4 to 6 ounces smoked tofu (depending on brand; some are more dense than others), cubed
	4 large iceberg lettuce leaves, washed and patted dry

Instructions

1. Fill medium saucepan with 1 inch of water. Place basket steamer in pan, and place green and yellow wax beans in steamer. Bring water to boil, cover, and steam beans until tender, about 4 to 5 minutes. Run beans under cold water to stop the cooking and retain color. Drain. Place in 2-quart mixing bowl and set aside.

2. In 1-quart saucepan combine onion, umeboshi vinegar, and brown rice or red wine vinegar. Cover and bring to boil. Remove from heat. Add olive oil, cover, and let stand 10 to 15 minutes. Add mustard, parsley, and garlic.

3. To the green or yellow beans, add garbanzo and kidney beans. Add seasoned onion mixture. Stir to coat. Add tofu and stir again. Arrange iceberg lettuce leaves on plate, and spoon bean and tofu mixture over lettuce.

Variation

Serve tofu on the side wrapped in lettuce leaves secured with toothpick.

Tuscan Tempeh and Chickpea Casserole with Broccoli

Servings: 1 Lunch or Dinner Entrée (4 blocks)

Block size	Ingredients
Tempeh mixture	
	1 tablespoon tamari soy sauce
	2-inch piece kelp sea vegetable, scissor-cut into cubes
	1 bay leaf + 1 cup purified water
1 carbohydrate, 4 protein	6 ounces plain soy tempeh, cubed
Sauté mixture	
4 fat	1⅓ teaspoons olive oil
¼ carbohydrate	1 cup mushrooms, thinly sliced
½ carbohydrate	½ cup onions, cut into thin half-ring slices
	1 clove garlic, minced or pressed
½ carbohydrate	¾ cup chopped or diced tomato, with juices
¼ carbohydrate	½ red or yellow bell pepper, cubed or cut in thin slices

	½ teaspoon each dried basil and oregano
	⅛ teaspoon ground red or black pepper
1 carbohydrate	¼ cup cooked, drained chickpeas
½ carbohydrate	2 cups broccoli, cut into florets, stems peeled and sliced finely
	Purified water for steaming

Instructions

1. Combine tamari, kelp, bay leaf, and water in a 1- to 1½-quart saucepan. Add tempeh cubes. Cover, bring to boil, then reduce heat and simmer without stirring for 30 minutes. Remove lid and simmer away liquid. Tempeh is ready to use now. Discard bay leaf. Chop kelp.

2. Add oil to 10-inch skillet. Heat, add mushrooms and onions. Stir until softened, reducing heat as needed to prevent scorching. Add garlic, diced tomato, bell pepper, spices, cooked tempeh, kelp pieces, and chickpeas. Bring to a boil, reduce heat to medium-low, cover, and simmer for about 20 minutes, until tender and liquid is reduced. Mixture should resemble a thick stew.

3. When tempeh casserole is almost done, place broccoli on a vegetable steamer tray over 1½ to 2 inches of boiling water in a medium-size sauce pan. Cover and steam for about 5 to 6 minutes or until broccoli is vibrant green and crisp-tender but not soggy or gray. Immediately transfer broccoli to a serving plate. Top with tempeh casserole. Serve.

Variation

After cooking tempeh, you may set one-fourth aside (one protein block worth) for tomorrow. Grate 1 ounce non-fat mozzarella cheese and sprinkle over tempeh casserole just before serving.

Greek Salad with Garlic-Oregano Dressing

Servings: 1 Lunch or Dinner Entrée (4 blocks)

Block size	Ingredients
1/2 carbohydrate	5 cups loosely packed romaine lettuce, washed, patted dry, torn into small pieces
1 carbohydrate	1 cup canned artichoke hearts, drained, cut into bite-size pieces
1 carbohydrate	2 medium tomatoes, cut into wedges
1/2 carbohydrate	1 small red onion, thinly sliced
1 carbohydrate	1/4 cup canned garbanzo beans, drained and rinsed
1 protein	2 ounces low-fat feta cheese, crumbled
3 protein	6 ounces extra-firm tofu, cut into 1/2-inch cubes
4 fat	1 1/3 teaspoons extra-virgin olive oil
	1 tablespoon red wine vinegar
	2 tablespoons vegetable stock or purified water
	1 small clove garlic, minced
	1/4 teaspoon dried oregano, crumbled
	1/4 teaspoon freshly ground black pepper

Instructions

1. Arrange lettuce on large dinner plate. Top with artichoke hearts, tomatoes, onions, garbanzo beans, feta cheese, and tofu.

2. In a small bowl, mix together olive oil, red wine vinegar, vegetable stock or water, garlic, oregano, and black pepper. Pour over salad and toss to evenly distribute dressing. Serve.

Variations

Replace half the lettuce with 1 large cucumber, peeled and diced.

Tempeh Taco Salad

Servings: 1 Lunch or Dinner Entrée (4 blocks)

Block size	Ingredients
Tempeh mixture	
	1 tablespoon tamari soy sauce
	2-inch piece kelp sea vegetable, scissor-cut into cubes
	1 bay leaf + 1 cup purified water
4 protein, 1 carbohydrate	6 ounces plain soy tempeh, cubed
Shell	
1 carbohydrate	1 (6-inch) corn tortilla
Sauté mixture	
2 fat	$2/3$ teaspoon olive oil
$1/4$ carbohydrate	$1/3$ cup onions, finely diced
$1/4$ carbohydrate	$1/2$ red or gold bell pepper, cut in small dice
	1 clove garlic, minced or pressed
	$1/4$ cup vegetable broth
	$1/2$ teaspoon ground cumin
	$1 1/2$ teaspoon chili powder
1 carbohydrate	$1/4$ cup cooked, drained black beans
Garnish	
$1/4$ carbohydrate	$2 1/2$ cups shredded green leaf or romaine lettuce
1 fat	1 tablespoon light sour cream
1 fat	3 olives, chopped
$1/4$ carbohydrate	$1/2$ cup cherry tomatoes, halved

Instructions

1. Combine tamari, kelp, bay leaf, and water in a 1- to 1$\frac{1}{2}$-quart saucepan. Add tempeh cubes. Cover, bring to boil, then reduce heat and simmer without stirring for 30 minutes. Remove lid and simmer away liquid. Discard bay leaf. Grate, mash, or mince tempeh and kelp finely.

2. Meanwhile, make slits on four outer edges of the tortilla. Place the tortilla inside a small heat-proof bowl, overlapping the edges to form to the sides of the bowl. Place the bowl on a cookie sheet and bake in a preheated 350°F oven until lightly crisped, about 5 to 10 minutes. Remove from oven. Allow to cool, then remove from bowl. Transfer to a bag and seal if made far ahead.

3. Add oil to a 10-inch skillet. Heat, add onions, bell pepper, and garlic. Stir until softened, about 2 to 3 minutes. Reduce heat to prevent scorching. Add vegetable broth and spices. Simmer for several minutes until liquid is absorbed. Remove from heat and add beans and tempeh mixture.

4. Spread 2 cups of lettuce on a dinner plate. Place taco bowl on top. Fill bowl with $\frac{1}{2}$ cup shredded lettuce. Top with tempeh-bean mixture, sour cream, olives, and tomato slices.

Variations

After cooking tempeh, set one-fourth aside (one protein block worth) for tomorrow. Grate 1 ounce non-fat mozzarella cheese and sprinkle over tempeh-bean mixture just before serving.

Replace tortilla baked in a bowl with one baked taco shell from a grocery or health food store.

Omit Step 1 above. Substitute 6-ounce portion of seasoned tempeh burgers. Mash or grate.

Tempeh Paprikas

Servings: 1 Lunch or Dinner Entrée (4 blocks)

Block size	Ingredients
Tempeh mixture	
	$1/2$ teaspoon sea salt **or** 1 tablespoon tamari
	4-inch piece kelp sea vegetable
	1 bay leaf + 1 cup purified water
	$1/4$ teaspoon ground cumin
	$1/8$ teaspoon ground black pepper
	$1/4$ teaspoon dried rosemary, crushed
4 protein, 1 carbohydrate	6 ounces plain soy tempeh, cubed
$1/2$ carbohydrate	2 cups cauliflower, cut into bite-size florets
1 carbohydrate	12 asparagus spears, cut into 2-inch lengths, bottom 1 inch discarded (about 1 cup sliced)
	Purified water to steam vegetables
	$1/4$ cup vegetable broth or purified water
1 carbohydrate	1 cup onion, cut into thin half-moons
	$1 1/2$ teaspoons ground paprika
$1/2$ carbohydrate	$1/2$ tablespoon arrowroot starch dissolved in $1/4$ cup cold purified water or vegetable broth
4 fat	4 tablespoons light sour cream or Nayonaise (tofu mayonnaise)

Instructions

1. Combine sea salt, kelp, bay leaf, water, spices, and herbs in a 1- to $1 1/2$-quart saucepan. Add tempeh cubes. Cover, bring to boil, then reduce heat and simmer without stirring for 30 minutes. Remove lid and simmer away liquid. Discard bay leaf. Reserve tempeh mixture for Step 3.

2. Scatter cauliflower over the bottom of a metal vegetable steamer. Arrange asparagus pieces on top. Rest steamer basket in a 2-quart saucepan filled with 1 to 2 inches of purified water. Just before serving, cover pot and bring to boil over medium heat. Steam vegetables for 5 to 8 minutes until just fork-tender. Immediately remove from heat and transfer to a dinner plate.

3. Add $1/3$ cup broth or water to a 9-inch skillet. Bring to boil, add onions, paprika, and cooked tempeh mixture from Step 1. Cover and bring to boil, reduce heat and simmer for about 5 to 6 minutes. Remove lid and add arrowroot mixture. Bring to boil, reduce heat to medium-low or low, and stir to thicken. Add sour cream or Nayonaise and stir until thick. If too thick, stir in 1 to 2 tablespoons water.

4. Spoon tempeh mixture over steamed vegetables and serve.

Variation

Replace 2 cups cauliflower with 2 cups green cabbage, cut into cubes or small wedges.

Mediterranean Tofu

Servings: 1 Lunch or Dinner Entrée (4 blocks)

Block size	Ingredients
4 fat	1$1/3$ teaspoons olive oil
$1/4$ carbohydrate	3 shallots, diced
	1 clove garlic, minced
4 protein	8 ounces extra-firm tofu, sliced into $1/2$-inch slices
1 carbohydrate	4 canned or jarred artichokes, drained, cut in half
$1/4$ carbohydrate	1 cup shiitake mushrooms, sliced
	$1/4$ cup white wine
	$1/4$ cup vegetable stock (recipe follows)
	$1/4$ teaspoon salt, or to taste
	Parsley sprigs for garnish
2$1/2$ carbohydrates	1$1/4$ cups fresh pineapple, cut into chunks

Instructions

1. Heat olive oil in medium sauté pan over medium heat. Add shallots and garlic. Cook, stirring constantly, until shallots and garlic turn translucent, about 2 to 3 minutes.

2. Add tofu and brown on both sides. Leave shallots and garlic in pan. Transfer tofu to plate. Cover to keep warm.

3. To pan, add artichokes and mushrooms. Cook about 5 minutes or until artichokes are heated through. Transfer to plate or bowl. Cover to keep warm.

4. Deglaze pan by adding white wine over medium heat. Lightly scrape bottom of pan with wooden spoon to release vegetable flavors. Add vegetable stock and salt and reduce liquid to a little over half.

5. Arrange tofu on plate. Top with vegetables and sauce. Garnish with parsley and serve. Serve pineapple for dessert.

Vegetable Stock

Lunch or Dinner stock—use in recipes as stock in place of chicken, veal, or beef stock.
Yield: Approximately 6 1/2 cups stock

Block size	Ingredients
2 carbohydrates	2 cups leeks
2 carbohydrates	2 cups carrots, chopped
1 carbohydrate	1 1/2 cups onion, coarsely chopped
1 carbohydrate	2 cups celery, coarsely chopped
3/4 carbohydrate	1 large zucchini, chopped
	1 bunch fresh parsley
	1/2 bunch fresh thyme
	7 whole peppercorns
	8 cups water

Instructions

1. Trim leeks by cutting away dark green ends and bulb. Cut in half and wash thoroughly. Coarsely chop.

2. Put all ingredients into a large stock pot. Bring to a boil, then simmer 1½ to 2 hours.

3. Strain through a fine sieve or strainer. Cool. Refrigerate or freeze and use as necessary.

Crazy for Curry, or Cauliflower Curry

Servings: 1 Lunch or Dinner Entrée (4 blocks)

Block size	Ingredients
4 fat	1⅓ teaspoons olive oil
	1 teaspoon cumin seed
	1 teaspoon mustard seed
	1 large clove garlic, minced
	1 to 2 inches fresh gingerroot, peeled and grated to equal 1 tablespoon
	Pinch freshly ground black pepper
	1 tablespoon curry powder (preferably Madras/hot)
4 protein	8 ounces extra-firm tofu, cut into cubes
1 carbohydrate	4 cups cauliflower florets
1 carbohydrate	1½ cups fresh green beans, cut into 1-inch pieces
	¼ cup vegetable stock (page 122)
2 carbohydrate	1 pear

Instructions

1. Heat oil in large sauté pan over medium heat.

2. Add cumin and mustard seeds and cook until coated. Add minced garlic, grated ginger, black pepper, and curry powder. Sauté for 1 minute to blend flavors.

3. Add tofu, cauliflower florets, beans, and vegetable stock. Cook, stirring occasionally, for 10 to 15 minutes or until cauliflower is tender. Serve immediately. Serve pear for dessert.

Vegetable and Tofu Kebabs

Servings: 1 Lunch or Dinner Entrée (4 blocks)

Block size	Ingredients
	4 to 6 wooden skewers, soaked in water overnight
4 protein	8 ounces extra-firm tofu, patted dry and cut into 1-inch cubes
1/2 carbohydrate	1 large red pepper, seeded and cut into large pieces
1/2 carbohydrate	1 large green pepper, seeded and cut into large pieces
1 carbohydrate	2 large red onions, cut into large pieces
1 carbohydrate	2 medium zucchini, cut into 1-inch slices
1 carbohydrate	2 medium summer squash, cut into 1-inch slices
4 fat	1 1/3 teaspoons olive oil (up to 1/2 cup)
	4 tablespoons dried thyme
	4 tablespoons dried oregano
	2 tablespoons garlic powder
	1 teaspoon salt
	1 teaspoon freshly ground black pepper

Instructions

1. Put tofu and vegetables on wooden skewers, being gentle with tofu so it doesn't break. Lay vegetable kebabs at bottom of shallow pan or bowl.

2. In a small bowl or jar, mix together olive oil, thyme, oregano, garlic powder, salt, and pepper. If need be, use up to $\frac{1}{2}$ cup olive oil for the marinade. Pour mixture over kebabs and let marinate, refrigerated, for at least $1\frac{1}{2}$ hours.

3. Prepare grill or broiler.

4. Place kebabs on grill, medium flame, turning frequently. Watch carefully so vegetables don't burn. Cook until vegetables are tender. Serve warm.

Black Beans al Fresco

Servings: 1 Lunch or Dinner Entrée (4 blocks)

Block size	Ingredients
4 fat	$1\frac{1}{3}$ teaspoons olive oil
	1 large clove garlic, minced
	1 tablespoon fresh parsley, chopped
	1 tablespoon fresh basil, chopped
	1 teaspoon dried rosemary
4 protein	8 ounces extra-firm tofu, cubed
4 carbohydrate	1 cup canned black beans, drained and rinsed
	3 tablespoons vegetable stock (page 122)
	1 teaspoon lemon juice, or to taste
	Pinch salt, or to taste
	Pinch freshly ground black pepper

Instructions

1. Heat oil in medium sauté pan over medium heat.

2. Add minced garlic, parsley, basil, and rosemary. Cook for 1 minute to blend flavors.

3. Add tofu and sauté until golden brown. Add black beans, vegetable stock, and lemon juice. Stir in salt and pepper. Taste and adjust seasoning.

4. Cook, stirring mixture, until heated through, about 5 to 10 minutes. Serve hot.

Garden "Sausage" Frittata

Servings: 1 Lunch or Dinner Entrée (4 blocks)

Block size	Ingredients
4 fat	1⅓ teaspoons olive oil
½ carbohydrate	1 medium onion, chopped
1 protein	2 links soy sausage, if frozen, thawed, and cut into ½-inch slices
1 carbohydrate	1½ cups fresh green beans, cut in ½-inch pieces
½ carbohydrate	1 large summer squash, diced
½ carbohydrate	1 large zucchini, diced
⅛ carbohydrate	¼ green bell pepper, diced
¼ carbohydrate	½ red bell pepper, diced
¼ carbohydrate	½ yellow bell pepper, diced
⅛ carbohydrate	½ cup button mushrooms
	½ teaspoon salt, or to taste
	Pinch freshly ground black pepper
3 protein	6 egg whites, extra large
¾ carbohydrate	⅓ cup blueberries, fresh

Instructions

1. Preheat oven to 400°F.

2. Heat oil in non-stick sauté pan that can go into oven. Add onion and cook until translucent, about 4 minutes.

3. Add sausage, green beans, summer squash and zucchini, bell peppers, and mushrooms. Season with salt and pepper. Sauté until tender, about 5 minutes. Remove from pan and set aside in bowl.

4. Whip egg whites until slightly foamy.

5. Add egg whites to pan over medium heat. Stir briskly with wooden spoon. Let cook over medium flame until bottom of egg whites set. Distribute vegetables evenly over partially cooked egg whites.

6. Remove pan from heat and place in oven until eggs are set, about 5 to 7 minutes.

7. Cut in quarters and serve immediately. Serve blueberries for dessert.

Spinach Omelet

Servings: 1 Lunch or Dinner Entrée (4 blocks)

Block size	Ingredients
4 fat	1¹/₃ teaspoons olive oil
1 carbohydrate	2 medium onions, chopped
	1 clove garlic, minced
	1 cup fresh spinach, cleaned and chopped
	¹/₄ teaspoon salt, or to taste
4 protein	8 egg whites, extra large
	Pinch freshly ground black pepper
3 carbohydrate	1 cup applesauce

Instructions

1. Heat oil in medium omelet or non-stick sauté pan with a cover over medium-low heat.

2. Add onion and garlic and cook until onions are translucent, about 5 minutes.

3. Add spinach and a pinch of the salt. Cook over medium heat until hot. Transfer to bowl or plate, cover to keep warm.

4. Whip egg whites until slightly foamy.

5. Pour egg whites into pan over medium heat. Sprinkle with remaining salt and pepper. Stir with wooden spoon and distribute egg evenly over pan.

6. Add spinach mixture to one side of eggs. Cover pan and cook over low heat for about 3 minutes or until egg is set.

7. Fold omelet in half and serve hot. Serve applesauce for dessert.

Citrus-Tofu Fennel Salad

Servings: 1 Lunch or Dinner Entrée (4 blocks)

Block size	Ingredients
2 carbohydrate	1 large fennel bulb
2 carbohydrate	1 orange
4 protein	8 ounces extra-firm tofu, patted dry and diced
	2 sprigs watercress, chopped
4 fat	1 1/3 teaspoons olive oil
	Juice of 1/2 lime
	Pinch of salt, or to taste

Instructions

1. Boil water in small saucepan. Cut fennel bulb in half, then thinly slice. Blanch fennel in boiling water. Remove and dunk into ice bath to cool. Drain.

2. Peel orange and section by cutting away thin membrane around segments. Retain juices and pulp in small bowl. Set aside.

3. In medium-size bowl, mix together tofu, fennel, orange segments, and watercress. Set aside.

4. To orange juice and pulp, add olive oil, lime juice, and salt. Toss tofu, fennel, and orange with dressing. Arrange on plate and serve.

Savory Lentils with Goat Cheese

Servings: 1 Lunch or Dinner Entrée (4 blocks)

Block size	Ingredients
4 carbohydrates	1 cup lentils, rinsed and drained
	1/2 teaspoon salt
	2 cups water
	1 clove garlic, minced
	2 tablespoons cilantro
	2 tablespoons chives, chopped
4 fat	1 1/3 teaspoons olive oil
	Juice of 1 lime
4 protein	4 ounces goat cheese, room temperature
	1/8 teaspoon freshly ground pepper, or to taste
	2 radicchio leaves for garnish

Instructions

1. In a medium saucepan, place lentils, 1/4 teaspoon of the salt, and water. Bring to a boil and simmer for about 20 minutes or until lentils are tender, but still have texture. Remove from heat and drain.

2. In a medium-size bowl, mix lentils, garlic, cilantro, and chives together. Add olive oil and lime juice. Toss gently.

3. Before serving, fold in goat cheese. Season with remaining salt and pepper. Arrange radicchio leaves on plate. Spoon salad onto radicchio and serve.

Note: Serve chilled, room temperature, or warm.

Black Bean Salsa

Servings: 4 blocks carbohydrate and 4 blocks fat only (see Note below)

Block size	Ingredients
3 carbohydrate	3/4 cup canned black beans, drained and rinsed
1 carbohydrate	1 1/2 cups tomato, diced
1/4 carbohydrate	1/2 small red onion, chopped
4 fat	1 1/3 teaspoons olive oil
	Juice of 1 lime
	4 tablespoons cilantro, chopped
	1/2 jalapeño pepper, or to taste
	Pinch of salt, or to taste
	Pinch of freshly ground pepper, or, to taste

Instructions

1. Mix black beans, tomato, red onion, olive oil, lime juice, and cilantro in a medium-size bowl.

2. Seed jalapeño pepper by cutting in half and taking out seeds. Since the heat of the pepper is mostly in the seeds, you may want to wear rubber gloves or be careful working with pepper. Finely chop half the pepper and add to mixture.

3. Add salt and pepper. Taste and adjust seasoning. For more "heat," cut remaining jalapeño pepper and add to salsa.

Note: This can be used as a condiment to Spinach Omelet or Frittata (page 127) or other proteins.

Red-Bean Chili

Servings: 1 Lunch or Dinner Entrée (4 blocks)

Block size	Ingredients
4 fat	1⅓ teaspoons olive oil
¼ carbohydrate	½ medium onion, chopped
¼ carbohydrate	½ medium green bell pepper, seeded and chopped
	1 teaspoon chili powder
	½ teaspoon ground cumin
	¼ teaspoon sea or regular salt
	¼ teaspoon garlic powder, or 1 clove garlic, chopped
2 protein	⅔ cup Morningstar Farms Harvest Burgers Recipe Crumbles (found in the freezer section, usually with the breakfast meats)
	½ cup water
1½ carbohydrate	1¼ cups canned crushed tomatoes
2 carbohydrate	½ cup canned kidney beans, drained and rinsed*
2 protein	2 ounces low-fat Monterey Jack or soy cheese, grated or thinly sliced

Instructions

1. In large non-stick sauté pan with cover, heat oil over medium heat. Sauté onions and green pepper in oil for 5 minutes or until onion turns translucent.

2. Add chili powder, cumin, salt, and garlic powder. Cook another 2 minutes.

3. Add Harvest Burgers and water. Stir in tomatoes and kidney beans. Cover and simmer 10 to 30 minutes to blend flavors.

4. Serve in a bowl and sprinkle with grated cheese.

Note: You can leave beans out of recipe and replace them with a side of fruit salad containing 2 blocks of carbohydrate.

Green Bean Nicoise

Serving: 1 Lunch or Dinner Entrée (4 blocks)

Block size	Ingredients
1½ carbohydrate	2¼ cups green beans, stemmed and washed
1 carbohydrate	¼ cup kidney or garbanzo beans, drained and rinsed
½ carbohydrate	1 tomato, quartered
4 fat	1⅓ teaspoons olive oil
	1 teaspoon cider vinegar
	1 teaspoon soy sauce
	1 clove garlic, chopped
	Pinch of salt
	Pinch of freshly ground pepper
2 protein	2 ounces low-fat feta cheese, crumbled
2 protein	2 ounces soy cheese, crumbled
1 carbohydrate	½ orange

Instructions

1. In a glass bowl, microwave green beans on high until desired firmness (8 to 12 minutes). When done, plunge into ice-cold water to cool. Drain and place in medium-size bowl.

2. Add kidney or garbanzo beans and quartered tomato to green beans. Set aside.

3. Combine oil, cider vinegar, soy sauce, garlic, salt, and pepper. Toss beans and tomato with vinaigrette.

4. On a medium-size plate, arrange the beans and tomato. Sprinkle with feta and soy cheeses. Serve chilled. Serve ½ orange for dessert.

Variation

Replace the feta cheese with 4 ounces extra-firm tofu, cubed.

Zoned Greek Salad

Servings: 1 Lunch or Dinner Entrée (4 blocks)

Block size	Ingredients
1/2 carbohydrate	5 cups loosely packed romaine lettuce, washed, spin-dried, and chopped into bite-size pieces
1 carbohydrate	1 can artichoke hearts, drained, cut into bite-size pieces
1 carbohydrate	2 cups cherry tomatoes, halved, **or** 2 medium tomatoes, cut into thin wedges or cubes
1/2 carbohydrate	1 medium red or white onion, cut into rings
1 carbohydrate	1/4 cup chickpeas
1 protein	1 ounce low-fat feta cheese, crumbled
3 protein	4 1/2 ounces seasoned, baked, firm tofu **or** 6 ounces plain, extra-firm tofu, cut into 1/2-inch cubes

Dressing	
4 fat	1 1/3 teaspoons extra-virgin olive oil
	1 tablespoon red wine vinegar
	2 tablespoons vegetable broth or purified water
	1 small clove garlic, minced or pressed
	1/4 teaspoon dried oregano, crumbled
	1/4 teaspoon ground black pepper
	Optional: pinch dulce flakes (sea vegetable flakes, available in natural foods store)

Instructions

1. Arrange lettuce on a large dinner plate or platter. Top with artichoke hearts, tomatoes, onion, chickpeas, feta cheese, and tofu.

2. Mix dressing ingredients in a small dish and drizzle over salad. Toss salad and serve.

Variations

Replace the feta cheese with 1 ounce of low-fat Colby, Monterey Jack, Romano, or provolone, grated.

Replace the feta cheese with an additional 2 ounces extra-firm, seasoned tofu.

Replace half of the lettuce with 1 cup peeled, diced cucumbers.

Ginger-Scallion Tofu Stir-Fry

Servings: 1 Lunch or Dinner Entrée (4 blocks)

Block size	Ingredients
1/2 carbohydrate	2 cups mushrooms, sliced
	1 tablespoon lite soy sauce
	1/8 cup vegetable stock (page 122)
	1 tablespoons fresh ginger, minced
	1 1/2 cloves garlic, minced
1 carbohydrate	1 1/2 cups tomatoes, chopped
4 protein	8 ounces extra-firm tofu, thinly sliced
4 fat	1 1/3 teaspoons canola oil
2 carbohydrate	3 cups snow peas, thawed if frozen
1/2 carbohydrate	1 1/2 cups scallions, cut into 1-inch pieces

Instructions

1. Combine mushrooms, soy sauce, vegetable stock, ginger, garlic, tomatoes, and tofu in a bowl and marinate 30 minutes.

2. Heat oil in a heavy skillet or wok over medium high heat.

3. Add tofu mixture and stir-fry 3 to 4 minutes.

4. Add snow peas and scallions and stir-fry 3 to 4 minutes or until snow peas are bright green.

Artichoke and Mushroom Ragout

Servings: 1 Lunch or Dinner Entrée (4 blocks)

Block size	Ingredients
4 fat	1 1/3 teaspoons canola oil
1 carbohydrate	4 cups mushrooms, sliced
	1/2 cup vegetable stock (page 122)
2 carbohydrate	2 cups canned peeled tomatoes, chopped
1 carbohydrate	1 cup canned artichoke hearts, chopped
	1/2 teaspoon oregano, dried and ground
	1/4 teaspoon thyme, dried and ground
	Salt and pepper to taste
	1 tablespoon parsley, minced
4 protein	8 ounces extra-firm tofu, cut into 1-inch slices

Instructions

1. Heat oil in a heavy, non-reactive saucepan over high heat. Sauté mushrooms 4 minutes or until lightly browned.

2. Add stock and boil until mixture is reduced by half. Add tomatoes, artichoke hearts, oregano, thyme, and salt and pepper to taste.

3. Simmer 4 minutes, stirring frequently, until sauce thickens. Stir in parsley and remove from heat. Set aside and keep warm.

4. Turn on broiler. Season tofu with pepper to taste. Arrange tofu on a broiler pan and broil 3–4 minutes per side or until tofu is golden. Serve tofu topped with sauce.

Grilled Pepper Tofu Steaks

Servings: 1 Lunch or Dinner Entrée (4 blocks)

Block size	Ingredients
4 fat	1$\frac{1}{3}$ teaspoons peanut oil
	1 tablespoon fresh ginger, grated
	$\frac{1}{4}$ cup mirin, or sweet rice wine
	2 tablespoons light tamari or lite soy sauce
2 carbohydrate	2 cups yellow onion, sliced in rings
4 protein	8 ounces extra-firm tofu, cut into 3-inch slices
2 carbohydrate	4 cups red and green bell peppers, cut into rings

Instructions

1. Combine all ingredients, except tofu and peppers, into a bowl. Mix thoroughly.

2. Add tofu and peppers and marinate 30 minutes.

3. While tofu mixture is marinating, preheat grill.

4. Remove tofu, peppers, and onions from marinade and reserve marinade.

5. Arrange tofu steaks, peppers, and onions on hot grill. Close cover and cook 2 minutes. Brush with marinade, close cover, and cook another minute.

Hong Kong Burger

Servings: 1 Lunch or Dinner Entrée (4 blocks)

Block size	Ingredients
4 fat	1$\frac{1}{3}$ teaspoons canola oil
4 protein	1$\frac{1}{3}$ cups Morningstar Farms Harvest Burgers Recipe Crumbles (found in the freezer section, usually with the breakfast meats)
	$\frac{1}{4}$ teaspoon fresh ginger, grated
	1 clove garlic, minced
$\frac{1}{2}$ carbohydrate	1$\frac{1}{2}$ cups cooked broccoli
$\frac{1}{2}$ carbohydrate	2 cups raw sliced mushrooms
2 carbohydrate	$\frac{2}{3}$ cup canned sliced water chestnuts
	1 tablespoon lime juice
	2 teaspoons Asian fish sauce
	$\frac{1}{8}$ teaspoon crushed red pepper
	2 red lettuce leaves
1 carbohydrate	1 cup red onion, thinly sliced
	$\frac{1}{4}$ scallion, chopped
	1 tablespoon fresh cilantro, chopped

Instructions

1. Heat canola oil in a heavy non-stick skillet over medium high heat. Sauté soy crumbles, ginger, garlic, broccoli, mushrooms, and water chestnuts 10 minutes, stirring often, until mixture is warmed throughout.

2. Stir in lime juice, fish sauce, and pepper. Bring to a boil and cook 1 to 2 minutes, until liquid is evaporated by half.

3. Arrange lettuce on a serving dish. Mound hot soy mixture in center.

4. Garnish with red onion, scallion, and cilantro.

Sicilian Soy Sauce

Servings: 1 Lunch or Dinner Entrée (4 blocks)

Block size	Ingredients
3 carbohydrate	1½ cups tomato sauce
4 protein	1⅓ cups Morningstar Farms Harvest Burgers Recipe Crumbles (found in the freezer section, usually with the breakfast meats)
1 carbohydrate	2 cups frozen sliced colored peppers
	Italian seasonings (garlic, onion, basil, oregano, etc.)
4 fat	1⅓ teaspoons extra-virgin olive oil

Instructions

1. Heat sauce in medium saucepan.

2. Add soy crumbles and peppers.

3. Add fresh or dried Italian seasonings to taste.

4. Cook at medium heat until done.

5. Sprinkle olive oil over dish just before removing from heat.

Pepper-Fried Soy Steak

Servings: 1 Lunch or Dinner Entrée (4 blocks)

Block size	Ingredients
	1/8 cup water
4 protein	1 1/3 cup Morningstar Farms Harvest Burgers Recipe Crumbles (found in the freezer section, usually with the breakfast meats)
1 carbohydrate	2 cups green bell pepper, chopped
2 carbohydrate	2 medium white onions, chopped
	1 teaspoon of seasoned salt (see Note)
1 carbohydrate	1 1/2 cups raw tomato, diced
4 fat	1 1/3 teaspoons olive oil

Instructions

1. Heat water to boil in medium saucepan.

2. Add soy crumbles.

3. Add peppers and onion.

4. Add seasoned salt to taste. Cook until all the water is gone (15 minutes).

5. Toss in diced raw tomato and olive oil.

6. Stir until warmed.

Note: Seasoned salt: 2 parts salt, 1 part onion powder, and 1 part pepper

Chili Cha-Cha

Servings: 1 Lunch or Dinner Entrée (4 blocks)

Block size	Ingredients
	1/2 cup water
1 carbohydrate	1 medium onion, finely chopped
1/2 carbohydrate	1 cup sliced celery
2 carbohydrate	1/2 cup light red kidney beans, canned
4 fat	1 1/3 teaspoons canola oil
4 protein	1 1/3 cups Morningstar Farms Harvest Burgers Recipe Crumbles (found in the freezer section, usually with the breakfast meats)
	1/2 teaspoon sugar (or sweetener of choice)
1/2 carbohydrate	1 cup tomatoes, chopped
	1/2 teaspoon ground marjoram
	1/4 teaspoon ground cumin
	1/4 chopped red sweet pepper
	1/4 tablespoon garlic, minced
	1/2 teaspoon cayenne pepper
	Salt and pepper to taste

Instructions

1   Heat water to boil in large pot.

2. Braise the onion and celery.

3. Add the beans, including the juice in the can.

4. Add the remaining ingredients.

5. Simmer for 30 minutes.

Soy Baked Cheese and Vegetables

Servings: 1 Lunch or Dinner Entrée (4 blocks)

Block size	Ingredients
2 fat	2/3 teaspoon olive oil
3 protein	1 cup Morningstar Farms Harvest Burgers Recipe Crumbles (found in the freezer section, usually with the breakfast meats)
1/2 carbohydrate	1/2 medium onion, chopped
1/4 carbohydrate	1/2 cup red bell pepper, seeded and chopped
	1 clove garlic, minced
1/2 carbohydrate	1 cup yellow squash, thinly sliced
	1/4 teaspoon Italian herb seasoning
	Salt and pepper to taste
2 fat	6 black olives, pitted and minced
3/4 carbohydrate	8 ounces Italian-style peeled tomatoes, drained and chopped
1 protein	1 ounce low-fat cheddar cheese or soy cheese, shredded
2 carbohydrates	2/3 cup unsweetened natural applesauce

Instructions

1. Preheat oven to 375°F.

2. Heat olive oil in a heavy ovenproof skillet or casserole over medium-high heat.

3. On stovetop, combine soy crumbles, onion, red pepper, and garlic in skillet or casserole. Cook 5 minutes, stirring often, until onions are translucent.

4. Add squash, Italian seasoning, and salt and pepper to taste. Cook about 5 minutes, stirring often, until squash is crisp-tender.

5. Spread olives and tomatoes on top of squash mixture and cover tightly. Bake 10 minutes. Uncover and bake about 20 minutes, until liquid in skillet is almost completely evaporated. Sprinkle cheese over top and bake about 5 minutes longer, until cheese melts.

6. Serve applesauce as a side dish.

Soyburger with Green Beans

Servings: 1 Lunch or Dinner Entrée (4 blocks)

Block size	Ingredients
4 fat	1⅓ teaspoons olive oil
3 protein	1 cup Morningstar Farms Harvest Burgers Recipe Crumbles (found in the freezer section, usually with the breakfast meats)
½ carbohydrate	½ medium onion, chopped
	1 clove garlic, minced
1 carbohydrate	1 cup canned chopped tomatoes
	1½ teaspoons tomato paste
	¼ teaspoon oregano
	¼ teaspoon ground allspice
	Salt and pepper to taste
½ carbohydrate	1 cup Delmonte canned green beans, drained
1 protein	3 teaspoons grated Parmesan cheese
2 carbohydrate	1 cup red seedless grapes

Instructions

1. Heat oil in a heavy non-stick skillet over medium-high heat.

2. Sauté crumbles, onion, and garlic about 5 minutes, stirring, until onions are translucent.

3. Stir in tomato paste, oregano, and allspice. Season with salt and pepper to taste and bring to a boil. Reduce heat to medium and simmer 5 to 10 minutes, or until liquid is reduced by half.

4. Stir in green beans and bring to a simmer. Sprinkle cheese over top and serve grapes on the side.

Cajun Salmon and Tofu

Servings: 1 Lunch or Dinner Entrée (4 blocks)

Block size	Ingredients
2 protein	4 ounces extra-firm tofu, cut into 1-inch slices
2 protein	3 ounces salmon filet, skinned, cut into 1-inch slices
	1½ cloves garlic, cut in half
	¾ teaspoon paprika
	¼ teaspoon seasoned salt
	½ teaspoon sage, crumbled
	¼ teaspoon cayenne pepper
	¼ teaspoon ground black pepper
4 fat	1⅓ teaspoons canola oil
	⅛ cup water
½ carbohydrate	1½ cups frozen broccoli florets
2 carbohydrate	½ cup canned kidney beans, rinsed
1½ carbohydrate	¾ cup green seedless grapes

Instructions

1. Rub both sides of tofu and salmon filet with garlic.

2. Combine paprika, seasoned salt, sage, cayenne pepper, and black pepper in a bowl.

3. Press seasoning mixture into tofu and salmon with hands to adhere.

4. Heat oil in a heavy non-stick skillet over high heat. Add salmon and tofu. Reduce heat to medium and cook 4 to 5 minutes per side or until tofu is golden and cooked throughout. Watch salmon closely. Salmon should be removed when the pieces are cooked through, most likely before the tofu is done.

5. In a small saucepan, bring water to a boil. Add frozen broccoli florets and kidney beans. Cook until broccoli is heated through (it will be bright green in color).

6. Arrange tofu, salmon, broccoli, and kidney beans on the plate. Serve grapes as dessert.

Salmon, Tofu, and Green Bean Salad

Servings: 1 Lunch or Dinner Entrée (4 blocks)

Block size	Ingredients
2 protein	3 ounces canned salmon, drained, broken into chunks, skin and large bones removed
2 protein	4 ounces extra-firm tofu, cut into 1-inch cubes
1/2 carbohydrate	1 cup frozen cut green beans, thawed
1/2 carbohydrate	3/4 cup onion, sliced, separated into rings
	1 clove garlic, minced
3 fat	1 1/2 tablespoons Kraft Creamy Italian dressing
	1/2 cup iceberg lettuce, shredded
1/2 carbohydrate	3/4 medium cucumber, peeled, seeded, and diced
1 carbohydrate	1/4 cup canned cooked chickpeas, rinsed
1/2 carbohydrate	1 medium tomato, cut into wedges
1 fat	1 teaspoon almonds, slivered
1 carbohydrate	1/3 cup canned unsweetened fruit cocktail (packed in water)

Instructions

1. Combine salmon, tofu, green beans, onion, and garlic in a bowl.

2. Pour salad dressing over tofu/salmon mixture and toss gently.

3. Optional: Refrigerate for 1 1/2 to 3 hours to blend flavors.

4. Serve on bed of shredded lettuce, cucumbers, and chickpeas. Garnish with tomato wedges. Sprinkle slivered almonds on top. Serve fruit cocktail as dessert.

Tofu-Swordfish Stir-Fry

Servings: 1 Lunch or Dinner Entrée (4 blocks)

Block size	Ingredients
	1 ounce mushrooms, chopped
	2 teaspoons lite soy sauce
	2 tablespoons vegetable stock (page 122)
	2 teaspoons fresh ginger, minced
	1½ cloves garlic, minced
¼ carbohydrate	⅓ cup onion, sliced in rings
1 carbohydrate	½ cup carrots, sliced
2 protein	4 ounces extra-firm tofu, thinly sliced
2 protein	3 ounces swordfish steak, cut into 1-inch cubes
4 fat	1⅓ teaspoon canola oil
½ carbohydrate	¾ cup snow peas, thawed if frozen
¼ carbohydrate	¾ cup scallions, cut into 1-inch pieces
2 carbohydrate	⅔ cup canned mandarin orange sections (canned in water)

Instructions

1. Combine mushrooms, soy sauce, vegetable stock, ginger, garlic, onion, carrots, tofu, and swordfish in a bowl and marinate 30 minutes.

2. Heat oil in a heavy skillet or wok over medium-high heat.

3. Add tofu/swordfish mixture and stir-fry 3 to 4 minutes. Add snow peas and scallions. Stir-fry 3 to 4 minutes or until carrots are tender.

4. Serve mandarin oranges as dessert.

Dinner Entrées

Baked Golden Tofu Dumplings
with Saucy Dip

Servings: 1 Dinner Entrée (4 blocks)

Block size	Ingredients
Dumplings	
4 protein	8 ounces extra-firm tofu
4 fat	4 teaspoons natural peanut butter
	1½ tablespoons tamari sauce
	3 scallions, chopped
½ carbohydrate	1 small green or red pepper, chopped
¼ carbohydrate	2 medium stalks celery, chopped
¼ carbohydrate	8 medium mushrooms, diced
¼ carbohydrate	3 water chestnuts, diced
	1 medium sprig parsley, minced
Sauce	
1¼ carbohydrate	³/₄ cup apple juice
1 carbohydrate	2 teaspoons maple syrup or brown sugar
	1 to 2 teaspoons tamari sauce
	1 to 2 teaspoons apple cider vinegar
	Optional: ½ teaspoon ginger, grated
	2 cloves garlic, pressed
	1 to 2 teaspoons arrowroot powder dissolved in 1 to 2 teaspoons water
½ carbohydrate	4 medium leaves kale, washed and de-stemmed

Instructions

1. Preheat oven to 375°F.

2. Mash tofu with fork or potato masher until broken up. Add peanut butter, tamari sauce, scallions, pepper, celery, mushrooms, water chestnuts, and parsley. Mix well.

3. Form the tofu mixture into golf ball-sized dumplings, and place on lightly oiled cookie sheet. Rinse hands in cold water periodically to keep dumplings from clinging.

4. Bake in oven for 30 minutes, or until golden brown.

5. Meanwhile, combine apple juice, maple syrup, tamari sauce, vinegar, ginger, and garlic in small saucepan. Bring to a simmer and cook for 1 to 2 minutes. Add arrowroot water and stir 1 minute more. Remove from heat.

6. Steam kale for 5 to 7 minutes.

7. Serve dumplings on a bed of steamed kale with a small dish of sauce on the side.

Barley-Mushroom Soup with Smoked Tofu

Servings: 1 Dinner Entrée (4 blocks)

Block size	Ingredients
2 carbohydrate	1 tablespoon barley
	4 cups vegetable stock (page 122)
4 fat	1⅓ teaspoons olive oil
½ carbohydrate	1 medium onion, chopped
¼ carbohydrate	2 medium stalks celery, chopped
¼ carbohydrate	8 medium mushrooms, sliced
½ carbohydrate	¼ cup tomato puree
4 protein	8 ounces smoked (or plain) extra-firm tofu, cubed
	1 medium spring parsley, minced
½ carbohydrate	1 medium ripe tomato, chopped

Salt and pepper to taste
Optional: vegetarian Worcestershire sauce,
    (available at health food stores)

Instructions

1. Combine barley and vegetable broth in medium stockpot, bring to a boil, and simmer for 20 minutes.

2. In separate pan, sauté olive oil, onion, and celery over medium-high heat for 4 to 5 minutes. Add mushrooms, increase heat to high, and brown for 3 to 4 minutes, until mushrooms release their juice.

3. Add sauté and tomato puree to barley broth. Simmer for 20 minutes. Add cubed tofu and simmer 5 minutes longer.

4. Serve in hefty bowls, topped with parsley, fresh tomato, salt, pepper, and vegetarian Worcestershire sauce.

Chunky Miso Soup

Servings: 1 Dinner Entrée (4 blocks)

Block size	Ingredients
2 carbohydrate	1 tablespoon barley
	4 cups water or vegetable stock (page 122)
4 fat	1 1/3 teaspoons toasted sesame oil
1/4 carbohydrate	1 small onion, chopped
1/4 carbohydrate	2 medium stalks celery, chopped
1/4 carbohydrate	6 medium mushrooms, sliced
	2 medium shiitake mushrooms, stems removed and sliced
1/4 carbohydrate	1/4 medium cabbage, shredded
	2 thin slices fresh ginger, peeled
	Optional: 6 to 8 green or wax beans

1 carbohydrate	¼ cup kidney beans, cooked
	4 tablespoons red barley miso paste
4 protein	8 ounces extra-firm tofu
	1 scallion, sliced

Instructions

1. Combine barley and water or broth in large pot, bring to a boil, and simmer covered for 20 minutes.

2. In separate pan, add sesame oil sauté onion and celery over medium heat for 3 to 4 minutes. Add mushrooms and cabbage and sauté 2 to 3 minutes more.

3. Add sauté, ginger, and green beans to barley broth and simmer covered for 20 minutes.

4. When ready to serve, remove 1 cup of broth from pot and stir into miso paste until smooth. Return broth and miso paste to the pot, remove from heat and stir gently. *Do not cook miso!* Cooking miso can destroy its beneficial properties. Add tofu and let stand for 2 to 3 minutes.

5. Stir once before serving in soup bowls. Garnish with scallion slices.

Easy Barbecue Tempeh and Vegetables

Servings: 1 Dinner Entrée (4 blocks)

Block size	Ingredients
4 fat	1⅓ teaspoons olive oil
¼ carbohydrate	½ small onion, diced
¼ carbohydrate	2 medium stalks celery, diced
	1 clove garlic, pressed
½ carbohydrate	1 red or green bell pepper, diced
2 protein, 2 carbohydrate	4 ounces tempeh, cubed
2 protein	⅓ cup TVP (textured vegetable protein)

	1/2 to 3/4 cup vegetable broth
	1 teaspoon prepared mustard
	1 teaspoon apple cider vinegar
	2 tablespoons barbecue sauce
1 carbohydrate	1/2 cup grapes

Instructions

1. Heat oil in large skillet and sauté onion and celery over medium-high heat until onions are translucent and slightly browned.

2. Add garlic, bell pepper, tempeh, and TVP and sauté 3 to 5 minutes longer. If the mixture starts sticking to skillet, add 2 to 3 tablespoons vegetable broth.

3. Add vegetable broth, mustard, vinegar, and barbecue sauce. Simmer covered about 20 minutes, until tempeh is infused with flavor.

4. Serve grapes for dessert.

Individual Baked Tofu Soufflés with Gravy and Roasted Vegetables

Servings: 1 Dinner Entrée (4 blocks)

Block size	Ingredients
Soufflé	
3 1/2 protein	7 ounces extra-firm tofu
1/2 protein	1 egg white
	3 teaspoons arrowroot powder
	1 tablespoon vegetable broth powder
	1/2 teaspoon salt
	3/4 teaspoon agar flakes
	1 tablespoon minced fresh rosemary
	(1 teaspoon if dried)

Roasted vegetables and gravy

4 fat	1$^{1}/_{3}$ teaspoons olive oil
1 carbohydrate	1 red bell pepper, roughly chopped
	1 green bell pepper, roughly chopped
$^{1}/_{2}$ carbohydrate	12 mushrooms, in chunks
$^{1}/_{2}$ carbohydrate	1 small red onion, roughly chopped
	1 medium sprig of parsley, minced
1 carbohydrate	1 tablespoon arrowroot powder dissolved in 1 tablespoon of water
	8 leaves fresh spinach
	$^{1}/_{2}$ orange

Instructions

1. Preheat oven to 375°F.

2. Combine tofu, egg white, arrowroot, broth powder, salt, agar, and rosemary in blender or food processor. Blend until creamy. Add 1 tablespoon of water at a time, if necessary, to help blend.

3. Spread with spoon or spatula into lightly oiled muffin tins. Create a cup about $^{1}/_{4}$ inch thick on the sides and the bottom.

4. Bake 30 minutes at 375°F. Remove from oven and let cool.

5. While cooling, combine oil with peppers, half the mushrooms, and half the onion in a roasting pan. Toss to coat with oil and lightly salt and pepper if desired. Cover and bake 15 minutes at 375°F. Uncover and bake 15 minutes longer. Broil the last 3 to 5 minutes, if desired, to crisp the vegetables.

6. Combine the rest of the mushrooms and onion in skillet to make gravy. Add fresh parsley and water to smooth consistency. Stir gently while cooking over high heat until bubbling. Add arrowroot water. Stir until well infused, about $^{1}/_{2}$ minute longer.

7. Remove soufflé cups from muffin tins and stand them upright. Fill cups with roasted vegetables, top with gravy, and serve on a bed of fresh spinach.

8. Serve orange for dessert.

Marinated Arame Sea Salad Slaw

Servings: 1 Dinner Entrée (4 blocks)

Block size	Ingredients
	Handful dried arame sea vegetable
2 fat	2 teaspoons tahini
	1 teaspoon umeboshi vinegar (Japanese plum vinegar)
	1/2 clove garlic, pressed
1/2 carbohydrate	Juice of 1/2 lemon
1 fat	1/3 teaspoon olive oil
4 protein	8 ounces extra-firm tofu, cubed
	1 tablespoon tamari or shoyu sauce
1 fat	1 teaspoon sesame seeds
1 carbohydrate	5 to 6 artichoke hearts, canned
1 carbohydrate	1/4 cup kidney beans
1 carbohydrate	1/4 cup black beans or chickpeas
1/2 carbohydrate	Juice of 1/2 lemon
	Salt and pepper to taste
	Optional: 1 small sprig parsley, minced
	Optional: 1/8 teaspoon garlic salt
	12 leaves fresh lettuce

Instructions

1. Cover arame in cold water, soak overnight in refrigerator. (QUICK TIP: For fast preparation, simmer for 10 to 15 minutes in water.) Drain, refresh with cold water, drain again. Chop arame coarsely.

2. Combine tahini, vinegar, garlic, lemon, and olive oil and whisk with a fork. Add arame, toss until coated, and refrigerate, if desired, until ready to assemble dish.

3. Toss tofu with tamari and sprinkle with sesame seeds. Set aside.

4. Combine artichoke, beans, lemon, and seasoning in a bowl. Set aside.

5. Lay out a thick bed of lettuce on each dinner plate. Place mound of arame in center. Encircle with tofu and artichoke and bean mixture.

Middle Eastern–Style Beans and Greens with Coriander

Servings: 1 Dinner Entrée (4 blocks)

Block size	Ingredients
1/2 carbohydrate	1 small onion, minced
4 fat	1 1/3 teaspoons olive oil
	1 clove garlic, pressed
	2 tablespoons fresh coriander (1 tablespoon if dried)
	1/4 teaspoon crushed hot red pepper
	1/2 teaspoon salt
	1/4 teaspoon allspice
1 carbohydrate	1/2 cup shelled fresh or frozen broad beans
3 protein	1 cup Morningstar Farms Harvest Burger Recipe Crumbles
	1 1/2 cups vegetable broth
1/2 carbohydrate	12 dandelion greens, washed and chopped fine
1/2 carbohydrate	Juice of 1/2 lemon
1/2 carbohydrate	1 medium tomato, chopped
1 protein	1 soy sausage patty
1 carbohydrate	1 plum

Instructions

1. Sauté onion in oil 5 to 7 minutes in skillet over medium-high heat. Add garlic, coriander, hot red pepper, salt, and allspice. Stir 1 to 2 minutes.

2. Add beans and soy crumbles and stir another 2 to 3 minutes until coated and warm.

3. Add vegetable broth. Cover and simmer on low heat until beans are tender, 25 to 30 minutes with fresh beans. (Cooking time with frozen beans will vary. See package for cooking time.)

4. Just as the beans are finishing, add dandelion greens, stir well, cover, and steam 5 to 7 minutes.

5. Serve piping hot topped with lemon juice and chopped tomato, and heated sausage patty on the side.

6. Serve plum for dessert.

Stir-Fry Tofu with Peppers and Peanuts

Servings: 1 Dinner Entrée (4 blocks)

Block size	Ingredients
1 fat	6 peanuts
3 fat	1 teaspoon peanut oil
4 protein	8 ounces extra-firm tofu, cubed
	1 clove garlic, pressed
	1/2 teaspoon fresh grated ginger
1 carbohydrate	3 turnip tops, washed and chopped coarsely
1/2 carbohydrate	1 1/3 tablespoons rice wine or sherry vinegar
1/2 carbohydrate	1 teaspoon pure maple syrup
	1 tablespoon tamari or shoyu sauce
	2 teaspoons arrowroot dissolved in 2 teaspoons water
	Optional: 1/2 teaspoon chili or Tabasco sauce
1/2 carbohydrate	1 small onion, diced
1 carbohydrate	1 small green bell pepper, diced
	1 small red bell pepper, diced
1/2 carbohydrate	12 mushrooms, sliced

1 clove garlic, pressed
1/2 teaspoon fresh ginger
2 scallions, sliced

Instructions

1. Roast peanuts in toaster oven or under broiler for 3 to 5 minutes, turning twice. Set aside.

2. Combine peanut oil and tofu in skillet and sauté over high heat. After 5 minutes, add garlic and ginger. Sauté another 3 minutes and remove from skillet.

3. Rinse and steam turnip tops in steamer basket over boiling water, or in small amount of water with no basket, until tender, about 10 minutes. Set aside with lid half off.

4. Mix rice wine vinegar, maple syrup, tamari, arrowroot, and Tabasco in a small bowl.

5. Combine onion, peppers, mushrooms, garlic, and ginger in a skillet and sauté 5 minutes on medium-high heat. Add water if necessary and stir regularly.

6. Stir up sauce in bowl and add to skillet. Stir until thickened. Add tofu and heat through, about 3 minutes.

7. Serve over bed of warm turnip tops. Top with peanuts and scallions.

Meatballs Parmigiana

Servings: 1 Dinner Entrée (4 blocks)

Block size	Ingredients
	Non-stick canola oil spray (to coat pan)
4 fat	12 walnut halves
2 protein, 1 1/2 carbohydrate	1/4 of a 14-ounce package of Gimme Lean, beef-style
1/2 protein	1 egg white
1/2 carbohydrate	1/2 tablespoon dried onion flakes

1 teaspoon dried parsley

$\frac{1}{2}$ teaspoon plus pinch of salt

$\frac{1}{2}$ teaspoon black pepper

$\frac{1}{4}$ teaspoon oregano

1 clove garlic, minced

Purified water

1 carbohydrate	$1\frac{1}{2}$ cups broccoli rabe (or regular broccoli)
1 carbohydrate	$\frac{1}{2}$ cup tomato sauce
$1\frac{1}{2}$ protein	$1\frac{1}{2}$ ounces part-skim mozzarella, shredded

Instructions

1. Preheat oven to 350°F.

2. Spray a baking sheet with non-stick canola oil spray. Set aside.

3. On another baking sheet, spread out walnut halves. Bake for 7 to 10 minutes, shaking or turning periodically to prevent burning, or until nuts are aromatic and lightly toasted. Cool. Place in blender container and blend to a coarse meal.

4. In medium bowl, combine ground walnuts, Gimme Lean, egg white, onion flakes, parsley, the $\frac{1}{2}$ teaspoon of salt, $\frac{1}{4}$ teaspoon of the black pepper, oregano, and garlic. Mix with potato masher until well blended. Form 1-inch balls and place on prepared baking sheet. Bake 10 minutes. Move balls around to coat with oil. Bake for another 10 to 12 minutes, or until golden brown and firm.

5. In a medium skillet with lid, add enough purified water to cover $\frac{1}{4}$ inch of pan. Add pinch of salt, rest of black pepper, and broccoli rabe. Bring to a boil. Cover and reduce heat to medium-low. Cook until tender.

6. Meanwhile, heat tomato sauce in small saucepan over medium heat.

7. When broccoli rabe is done, remove from heat. Arrange on serving plate. Top with meatballs and sauce, then sprinkle with mozzarella. Serve.

Orange, Tofu, and Spinach Salad

Servings: 1 Dinner Entrée (4 blocks)

Block size	Ingredients
1/4 carbohydrate	1 pound package pre-washed baby spinach or flat leaf spinach, stemmed, washed, spun dry, torn into large pieces
1/4 carbohydrate	1/2 grated carrot
1/2 carbohydrate	1/2 Walla Walla Sweet or Vidalia onions, cut into thin rings
2 carbohydrate	1 seedless orange, peeled and sectioned, **or** 2/3 cup mandarin orange sections
1 carbohydrate	1/3 cup water chestnuts, drained
4 protein	4 1/2 to 6 ounces smoked tofu, cubed
	1-inch piece of fresh gingerroot
	1/2 tablespoon umeboshi plum vinegar (*not* the same as regular vinegar— umeboshi is salty and tangy)
	1 tablespoon purified water
4 fat	1 1/3 teaspoons untoasted sesame or almond oil

Instructions

1. Place spinach in a large serving bowl. Top with grated carrot, onion rings, orange sections, water chestnuts, and tofu cubes.

2. Wash gingerroot and peel with paring knife or vegetable peeler. Grate on the smallest hole of a standard grater or use special ginger grater. Grab pulp. Make fist and squeeze over a small bowl or tablespoon. Wet pulp with a few drops of water, squeeze again, then discard pulp.

3. Combine ginger juice, umeboshi plum vinegar, water, and oil. Whisk with a fork. Pour over salad and toss with two large salad forks or spoons until salad wilts slightly. Transfer to a large salad plate and serve.

Variation

Replace tofu with 1 hard-boiled egg or 2 hard-boiled egg whites and 3 ounces of cubed skim or part skim cheddar, Colby, or other cheese. Prepare as above.

Ratatouille with "Sausage"

Servings: 1 Dinner Entrée (4 blocks)

Block size	Ingredients
4 fat	1⅓ teaspoons olive oil
¼ carbohydrate	⅓ cup onion, chopped
	½ teaspoon finely ground sea salt
	1 clove garlic, minced or pressed
¼ carbohydrate	½ cup peeled, diced eggplant
½ carbohydrate	1 cup zucchini, cut in half lengthwise, then cut into ½-inch-wide slices
¼ carbohydrate	½ gold or red bell pepper, seeded, diced
1 carbohydrate	½ cup bottled or canned unsweetened, oil-free tomato sauce **or** 1½ cups chopped, fresh tomato
	¼ teaspoon ground black pepper
	¼ teaspoon each dried basil, oregano, and thyme, crumbled between your fingers
1½ protein, 1 carbohydrate	2 Light Life Lean Links, cubed
¼ carbohydrate	1 cup cauliflower, cut into bite-size florets
	Purified water to steam
¾ carbohydrate	½ cup asparagus, sliced into 1-inch lengths
Topping	
2½ protein	2½ ounces low-fat mozzarella, cheddar, or Colby-style soy cheese, grated

Instructions

1. Add oil to a 1-quart saucepan or deep skillet. Heat to medium setting. Add onions, then sea salt. Stir and cook for about 3 minutes, until tender. Add garlic, eggplant, zucchini, and bell pepper, stirring after each addition. Cook for about 2 to 3 minutes. Add tomato sauce, pepper, basil, oregano, and thyme. Top with sliced "sausages" but do not stir. Cover, reduce heat to medium-low, and simmer for about 15 minutes, until vegetables are tender.

2. Meanwhile, place cauliflower on a metal vegetable steamer rack in a 2-quart pot filled with 1 to 2 inches of purified water. Top with asparagus. Cover and bring to boil over medium-high heat. Reduce heat to medium and steam for 5 to 7 minutes or until vegetables are fork-tender. Transfer cauliflower and asparagus to a large soup bowl or dinner plate with sides.

3. Remove lid from ratatouille and continue cooking for another 5 minutes to reduce liquid. Sprinkle with grated soy cheese and remove from heat. Serve ratatouille over steamed vegetables.

Note: Make a double batch to serve two people, or one person two days in a row. (If making a larger batch, add the cheese to individual portions at the table.) Store the leftovers in a jar, then reheat the next day.

Variation

Omit sausages, then increase soy cheese to 4 ounces.

Mexican-Style Summer Squash with Beans and Soy Cheese

Servings: 1 Dinner Entrée (4 blocks)

Block size	Ingredients
1/4 carbohydrate	1/3 cup + 1 tablespoon onion, chopped finely
	1/4 teaspoon finely ground sea salt
	1 clove garlic, minced or pressed
1/2 carbohydrate	1 cup zucchini, cut in half lengthwise, then in 1/2-inch rounds
1/2 carbohydrate	1 cup yellow summer squash, cut in half lengthwise, then in 1/2-inch rounds
1/4 carbohydrate	1/2 red bell pepper, seeded, quartered, cut in thin strips
	1/2 to 1 teaspoon chili powder (according to taste)
	1/4 teaspoon ground cumin
	1/4 teaspoon dried basil, crumbled
	1/4 teaspoon dried oregano, crumbled
	1 teaspoon tamari soy sauce
2 carbohydrate	1/2 cup cooked, drained black or red beans
4 protein	4 ounces non-fat mozzarella, Monterey Jack, or Colby-style soy cheese, grated

Salad

Block size	Ingredients
1/4 carbohydrate	2 1/2 cups shredded spring salad mix or red or green leaf lettuce
1/4 carbohydrate	1/2 cup cherry tomatoes, cut into half

Dressing

	2 to 3 teaspoons apple cider vinegar or lime juice

	1 teaspoon tamari or ume/umeboshi vinegar
	1/8 teaspoon ground red pepper
	1/4 teaspoon dry mustard (powder)
2 fat	2/3 teaspoon extra-virgin or virgin olive oil
1 fat	1 tablespoon light sour cream or Nayonaise
1 fat	3 olives, chopped

Instructions

1. Spray a non-stick 9- to 10-inch skillet with cooking spray, add onion and sauté. When onions begin to soften, add sea salt to draw out moisture. Add garlic, zucchini, summer squash, and bell pepper, stirring for 1 to 2 minutes after each addition. Add spices and tamari. (If using an electric range, you may need to add about 2 tablespoons of water to prevent sticking and burning.)

2. Cover skillet and bring to steam over medium-high heat. Reduce heat and simmer for 15 to 18 minutes, until vegetables are almost tender and juicy. Top with beans but do not stir. Cover and simmer for 4 to 5 minutes. Sprinkle cheese on top. Turn off and remove pan from heat source.

3. Arrange salad greens or lettuce and tomatoes on a large dinner plate. Mix dressing ingredients, then pour over salad. Transfer summer squash and beans dish to dinner plate and serve.

Southwestern Tofu over Black Beans

Servings: 1 Dinner Entrée (4 blocks)

Block size	Ingredients
4 protein	8 ounces extra-firm tofu, frozen in package, then thawed (this gives added texture to tofu)
1/2 carbohydrate	6 tablespoons mesquite marinade (see Note)

4 fats	1⅓ teaspoons olive oil
	½ small onion, chopped
	1 clove garlic, chopped
	1 teaspoon ground cumin
	¼ teaspoon sea or regular salt
2½ carbohydrate	½ cup plus ⅛ cup canned black beans, drained and rinsed
1 carbohydrate	¼ cup frozen corn
	One 10-ounce package frozen spinach, thawed and drained
	1 tablespoon lime juice
	1 to 2 tablespoons water

Instructions

1. Turn on broiler.

2. Cut thawed tofu into 1-inch slices and lay in 9 by 12-inch glass Pyrex dish. Cover both sides of tofu with marinade. Broil one side until browned. Turn and brown other side. Set aside.

3. Heat olive oil in medium non-stick sauté pan. Add onion, garlic, cumin, and salt. Cook for 2 to 3 minutes or until onion is translucent.

4. Add black beans, corn, spinach, lime juice, and water. Cook an additional 10 minutes or until all ingredients are heated through. Add extra salt if needed.

5. Arrange bean mixture on a plate, top with tofu, and serve.

Note: Mesquite marinade can be found in the barbecue section of your grocery store. Look on the label to find one that lists 1 gram carbohydrate per tablespoon serving.

Spinach Feta Pie

Servings: 4 Dinner Entrées (16 blocks)

Block size	Ingredients
12 fats	4 teaspoons olive oil
1 carbohydrate	1 large onion, chopped
1 carbohydrate	2 medium red bell peppers, chopped
4 fats	12 black olives, pitted and quartered
1 carbohydrate	6 10-ounce packages frozen chopped spinach, thawed and drained
	2 teaspoons garlic powder
	1 teaspoon sea or regular salt
1 protein	1 large whole egg
15 protein	15 ounces low-fat feta or soy cheese
4 carbohydrate	1 1/3 cups old-fashioned rolled oats
4 carbohydrate	8 high-fiber crackers, such as Kavli or Wasa
4 carbohydrate	1 medium cantaloupe, cut into 4 wedges or 2 grapefruits, halved

Instructions

1. Preheat oven to 350°F.

2. In a large non-stick sauté pan, heat the oil over medium heat. Add onions, red peppers, olives, spinach, garlic powder, and salt. Cook until heated through and most of the water is evaporated.

3. In a large bowl, beat egg and crumble in feta. Add spinach mixture and set aside.

4. To make crust, put rolled oats in blender or food processor with steel blade and pulse to create coarse oats. (Be careful not to overblend into a fine powder.)

5. Add 1/3 cup of the ground oats to spinach mixture. Spread remaining oats into bottom of 9 by 12-inch Pyrex dish or large pie plate. Evenly distribute spinach and cheese mixture over oats.

6. Bake for approximately 45 minutes or until pie is firm to the touch. Cut into 4 servings. Serve with crackers and fruit.

Stuffed Cabbage

Servings: 1 Dinner Entrée (4 blocks)

Block size	Ingredients
	5 medium-sized cabbage leaves, rinsed
3 fat	1 teaspoon olive oil
1/2 carbohydrate	1 medium onion, minced
1 fat	3 black olives, pitted and finely chopped
1/2 carbohydrate	1/2 tablespoon raisins, finely chopped
	1/4 teaspoon paprika
	1/4 teaspoon garlic powder, **or** 1 clove garlic, minced
	1/4 teaspoon sea or regular salt
	1/8 teaspoon black pepper
4 protein	8 ounces extra-firm tofu, drained and crumbled
1 carbohydrate	1/2 cup tomato sauce
2 carbohydrate	2/3 cup unsweetened applesauce

Instructions

1. In a covered glass bowl, microwave cabbage leaves in 1 tablespoon water for 4 minutes or until desired texture. Set aside to cool.

2. Heat oil in sauté pan over medium heat. Sauté onion, olives, and raisins for approximately 5 minutes or until onion turns translucent. Add paprika, garlic powder, salt, and pepper. Cook another 2 minutes.

3. Add tofu and 2 tablespoons of tomato sauce. Cook another 5 minutes.

4. Wrap filling in cabbage leaves. Serve with remaining tomato sauce.

5. Serve applesauce for dessert.

Tofu-Eggplant Gumbo

Serving: 1 Dinner Entrée (4 blocks)

Block size	Ingredients
4 fat	1 1/3 teaspoons olive oil
4 protein	8 ounces extra-firm tofu
	Celery salt, to taste
1 carbohydrate	1 1/2 cups onion, chopped
1/2 carbohydrate	1 cup green bell pepper, chopped
1/2 carbohydrate	1 cup celery, sliced
1 carbohydrate	1 cup tomato, crushed
1 carbohydrate	1 1/2 cups eggplant, peeled and diced
	2 cups vegetable stock (page 122) or bouillon
	2 teaspoons garlic, chopped
	1/2 teaspoon dried thyme
	1/8 teaspoon cayenne pepper
	1/4 cup fresh parsley, chopped
	Optional: salt and pepper to taste

Instructions

1. In a medium non-stick sauté pan, heat 2/3 teaspoon oil. Add tofu and sprinkle with celery salt. Stir-fry over medium-high heat until browned and crusted on all sides, about 5 minutes. Transfer browned tofu to a platter, lightly cover with aluminum foil to keep warm and set aside.

2. Heat remaining oil a 10- to 12-inch skillet. Add onion, peppers, celery, tomato, and eggplant. Add stock, garlic, and remaining spices except the salt and pepper and bring to a boil. Reduce heat and cook, covered, stirring occasionally until vegetables are almost tender, about 10 minutes. Add salt and pepper to taste.

3. Remove cover and continue cooking over high heat until liquid thickens and vegetables are tender, about 5 minutes more.

4. Spoon gumbo into a shallow soup bowl and top with tofu.

Cheese and Veggie Melt

Servings: 1 Dinner Entrée (4 blocks)

Block size	Ingredients
	3 to 4 tablespoons purified water (less for a gas range, more for electric)
	1 clove garlic, minced or pressed
	1/2 teaspoon dried basil, oregano, thyme, or combination
	Optional: 1/8 teaspoon ground black pepper
1/2 carbohydrate	1/2 cup onions, cut in half-ring slices
1/2 carbohydrate	1 cup red or yellow bell pepper, halved, seeded, cut in strips or 1-inch dice
1/3 carbohydrate	1 1/3 cups cremini or button mushrooms, sliced thin
1/3 carbohydrate	1 cup broccoli, cut in florets, stems peeled, cut thin
1/3 carbohydrate	1 1/3 cups cauliflower, cut into florets
1 carbohydrate	1/2 cup carrots, cut in thin rounds or half-moons
4 protein	4 ounces low-fat mozzarella, Colby, Monterey Jack, munster, or cheddar-style soy cheese, grated or cut in thin strips
4 fat	4 macadamia nuts or 12 almonds, raw or lightly toasted, coarsely chopped
1 carbohydrate	1/2 cup grapes

Instructions

1. Add water, herbs, and spices to an 8- or 9-inch skillet with a lid. If cooking for two, use two small skillets or one 10- to 12-inch skillet; for four people, use a 12- to 13-inch skillet.

2. Add vegetables to skillet in the order listed. Cover and bring to boil. Reduce heat and simmer for about 4 to 6 minutes, or until almost tender.

3. Meanwhile, weigh cheese unless it comes in 1-ounce logs (as with string cheese). Grate cheese. Remove lid from skillet; sprinkle nuts, then cheese over vegetables. Cover and simmer for 2 to 3 minutes or until cheese melts. Or sprinkle on cheese, then cover and turn off heat.

4. Remove from heat. Use a spatula to transfer vegetables and cheese to a dinner plate. Serve immediately. Serve grapes for dessert.

Curried Soy Cheese and Veggie Melt

Servings: 1 Dinner Entrée (4 blocks)

Block size	Ingredients
	3 to 4 tablespoons purified water (less for a gas range; more for electric)
	1 clove garlic, minced or pressed
	1/4 teaspoon ground turmeric
	1/2 to 1 teaspoon curry powder (or less the first time)
	Optional: 1/8 teaspoon ground black or white pepper
1/2 carbohydrate	1/2 cup onions, cut in rings or half-ring slices
1 carbohydrate	1 cup sliced zucchini or summer squash
1/4 carbohydrate	1 cup cauliflower, cut into florets
1 carbohydrate	1 1/2 cups green beans or yellow wax beans, ends trimmed, cut in 2-inch pieces
1/4 carbohydrate	1/2 cup red, yellow, or green bell pepper, halved, seeded, cut in strips or 1-inch dice
1 carbohydrate	1/4 cup frozen green peas

4 protein	4 ounces low-fat mozzarella, Colby, Monterey Jack, munster, or cheddar-style soy cheese, finely grated or cut in strips
4 fat	12 teaspoons walnut or pecan halves, coarsely chopped

Instructions

1. Add water and spices to an 8- or 9-inch skillet with a lid. If cooking for two, use two small skillets or one 10- to 12-inch skillet; for four people, use a 12- to 13-inch skillet.

2. Wash vegetables and chop. Add vegetables to skillet in the order listed. Cover and bring to boil. Reduce heat and simmer for about 4 to 6 minutes, or until almost tender.

3. Meanwhile, weigh soy cheese. Grate or chop finely. Remove lid from skillet; sprinkle "cheese" on top, then nuts. Cover and simmer for 2 to 3 minutes or until "cheese" melts.

4. Remove from heat. Use a spatula to transfer vegetables and cheese to a dinner plate. Serve immediately.

Apple Kanten with Maple Tofu Cream

Servings: 4 Dinner Desserts (1 block each)

Block size	Ingredients
Kanten	
3 carbohydrate	1 cup apple juice
	1 teaspoon pure vanilla extract
	(non-alcohol, glycerine base)
	1 tablespoon agar flakes
Tofu cream	
4 protein	8 ounces extra-firm tofu, blanched
4 fat	1⅓ teaspoons almond butter
1 carbohydrate	2 teaspoons sugar
	½ teaspoon pure vanilla extract
	(non-alcohol, glycerine base)
	1 teaspoon maple extract

Instructions

1. Combine apple juice, vanilla, and agar flakes in small saucepan and simmer for 5 minutes, stirring occasionally until agar dissolves.

2. Pour into dessert dish (or individual dessert dishes), leaving about ½ inch for the tofu cream topping.

3. Combine tofu, almond butter, sugar, vanilla, and maple extract in blender. Process on medium until smooth. Add 1 or 2 tablespoons of apple juice if necessary to help the ingredients blend.

4. Top kanten with tofu cream, chill, and serve.

Crunchy Top Peaches 'n' Cream

Servings: 4 Dinner Desserts (1 block each)

Block size	Ingredients
1 carbohydrate	1/3 cup rolled oats
1 fat	3 cashews, chopped
1 fat	1 macadamia nut, chopped
2 fat	6 almonds, chopped
2 carbohydrate	4 teaspoons pure maple syrup
4 protein	4 ounces skim ricotta cheese
	1/2 tablespoon pure vanilla extract (non-alcohol, glycerine base)
	1/2 tablespoon orange extract (non-alcohol, glycerine base)
	1 teaspoon cinnamon
1 carbohydrate	1 medium peach, washed and sliced

Instructions

1. In a dry skillet, gently roast oats, cashews, macadamia nut, and almonds over medium heat. Stir to keep from burning. Mix in 2 teaspoons maple syrup and remove from heat.

2. In a separate bowl, beat ricotta vigorously with vanilla and orange extracts, cinnamon, and remaining 2 teaspoons maple syrup. Mixture will start out curd-like. Beat by hand or with mixer until smooth and creamy.

3. Spoon ricotta onto chilled plate and top with peach slices and oat/nut crunch.

Lemon Meringue

Servings: 4 Dinner Desserts (1 block each)

Block size	Ingredients
Lemon filling	
2 carbohydrate	$2/3$ cup apple juice
$1/2$ carbohydrate	Juice of $1/2$ lemon
	$1/2$ tablespoon agar flakes
	1 teaspoon lemon extract
	(non-alcohol, glycerine base)
$1/2$ carbohydrate	1 teaspoon sugar
	1 teaspoon arrowroot powder dissolved in
	1 teaspoon water
2 protein	4 ounces extra-firm tofu
Meringue	
2 protein	4 egg whites, at room temperature
	$1/4$ teaspoon cream of tartar
1 carbohydrate	2 teaspoons sugar

Instructions

1. Preheat over to 400°F.

2. Combine apple juice, lemon, agar, lemon extract, and sugar in a small saucepan and simmer until agar dissolves, about 5 minutes. Remove from heat and add arrowroot, stirring constantly until it disappears.

3. Pour sauce into blender, add tofu, and blend until smooth. Pour into small ovenproof dish or miniature pie plate. Put aside to set.

4. Beat egg whites with cream of tartar until stiff. Add sugar and beat a moment longer.

5. Pile the meringue onto lemon filling and bake at 400°F for 5 to 7 minutes until golden.

Nectarine Freeze

Servings: 4 Dinner Desserts (1 block each)

Block size	Ingredients
	1 tablespoon agar flakes
2 carbohydrate	2/3 cup apple or orange juice
1 carbohydrate	1/2 ripe nectarine
1 carbohydrate	2 teaspoons sugar
4 protein	8 ounces extra-firm tofu
4 fat	4 macadamia nuts, chopped

Instructions

1. Simmer agar in juice until dissolved, about 5 minutes.

2. Combine dissolved agar, nectarine, sugar, tofu, and nuts in blender and blend until smooth. Place in freezer and chill until cold but not quite frozen. Serve in small chilled bowls.

Cinnamon Peaches with Ricotta

Servings: 4 Desserts (1 block each)

Block size	Ingredients
3 carbohydrate	3 fresh peaches, halved and pitted
	Scant $1/8$ teaspoon finely ground sea salt
1 carbohydrate	2 teaspoons fructose powder
	$1/4$ teaspoon ground cinnamon
4 protein	4 ounces part-skim ricotta, chilled
	2 teaspoons pure vanilla extract
	(non-alcohol, glycerine base)
4 fat	12 almonds, coarsely chopped

Instructions

1. Preheat broiler. Meanwhile, arrange peach halves, hollow side up, in a shallow baking pan. Sprinkle each half with sea salt, fructose powder, and cinnamon.

2. Place pan under broiler and cook until lightly brown, anywhere from 4 to 8 minutes.

3. In a small bowl, mix ricotta and vanilla extract. When peaches are done, scoop small mounds of ricotta into peach halves, distributing evenly. Sprinkle with nuts and serve.

Variations

In place of peaches, use other Zone blocks of fruits: one whole pear, halved; one nectarine, halved, plus $2/3$ cup raspberries; 9 apricots, halved; $1 1/2$ cups fresh pineapple, cut into bite-size chunks. Grill rather than broil fruit until tender.

Zoned Strawberry Ice Cream

Servings: 4 Snacks or Desserts (1 block each)

Block size	Ingredients
2 carbohydrate	$^2/_3$ cup almond or vanilla Amasake, chilled
2 carbohydrate	2 heaping cups frozen strawberries
	$^1/_4$ cup purified water
4 fat	2 teaspoons unsweetened almond butter
4 protein	$1^1/_3$ ounces plain, unflavored protein powder
	2 teaspoons pure vanilla extract (non-alcohol, glycerine base)
	$^1/_4$ teaspoon stevia extract powder

Instructions

1. Prepare ice cream maker per manufacturer's instructions. If the canister requires freezing, wrap in plastic bag and freeze for at least 24 hours. If ice and salt are required, have these ready. (Some models work best when they're at least half-full. You may need to prepare a double batch to use the machine effectively.)

2. Shake bottle of Amasake thoroughly. Measure out $^2/_3$ cup and add to blender container. Add strawberries, water, almond butter, protein powder, vanilla extract, and stevia. Cover and blend until smooth. Scrape down sides with spatula to incorporate all ingredients.

3. Start ice cream machine and pour in mixture. Freeze according to manufacturer's instructions. Portion into four serving bowls and serve.

Note: You can make ice cream mixture ahead of time and refrigerate overnight.

Variations

For blueberry ice cream, replace strawberries with 1 cup fresh blueberries.

If you don't own an ice cream maker, omit $1/4$ cup purified water. Blend all ingredients until smooth. Add 4 to 6 ice cubes through top feeder and blend on crush-ice mode until smooth and thick. Serve right away or freeze at least 3 to 4 hours in four single-serving containers. Allow to soften at room temperature for 10 minutes before serving.

Berries with Chocolate Almond Cream

Servings: 4 Snacks or Desserts (1 block each) or 1 Breakfast Entrée (4 blocks)

Block size	Ingredients
1 carbohydrate	1 cup "original" flavored almond milk (Pacific Foods of Oregon is a well-known brand)
	2 tablespoons agar flakes (vegan equivalent of gelatin, found in natural foods stores)
	2 rounded teaspoons unsweetened cocoa powder
4 protein	$1^{1}/3$ ounces unflavored soy protein powder (portion containing 28 grams protein)
4 fat	4 teaspoons unsweetened almond, hazelnut, or pistachio butter
	1 tablespoon pure vanilla or maple extract (non-alcohol, glycerine base)
	$1/2$ teaspoon stevia extract powder
	$1/4$ cup purified water
3 carbohydrate	3 cups fresh strawberries or raspberries, **or** 3 heaping cups frozen strawberries or raspberries, thawed

Instructions

1. Pour almond milk into a 1-quart saucepan and sprinkle agar flakes on top. Bring to boil over medium heat. Reduce heat and simmer for 5 minutes until agar is dissolved and mixture is smooth. Stir periodically with a wooden spoon.

2. Pour almond milk mixture into a blender. Cover and blend for 30 seconds. Add cocoa powder, protein powder, nut butter, vanilla, and stevia powder. Blend until smooth. Scrape down the sides of the blender with a spatula as needed to incorporate the powder.

3. Pour mixture into 12-ounce bowl. Chill for 2 to 3 hours or until firm to the touch.

4. Cut mixture into pieces with a large spoon and put back in the blender. Blend until smooth and creamy. Add water only as needed to blend. Chill again.

5. Combine fresh fruits in a large soup bowl or 4 wine goblets. Top with nut cream.

Variation

Replace 1 cup strawberries or raspberries with $\frac{1}{2}$ cup blueberries or grapes or $\frac{3}{4}$ cup cantaloupe or boysenberries.

"Cream" of Zucchini Soup

Servings: 4 Appetizers (1 block each)

Block size	Ingredients
4 fat	1⅓ teaspoons olive oil
½ carbohydrate	½ cup onion, cut into thin rings or half-moons
1½ carbohydrate	3 cups zucchini, diced
	1 clove garlic, minced or pressed
	2 cups purified water
2 protein	¼ cup soy flour
	3 tablespoons nutritional yeast flakes
	½ teaspoon dried dill weed **or** ¼ teaspoon ground nutmeg
1 carbohydrate	2 tablespoons white, yellow, or sweet light miso (not red, barley, buckwheat, or dark miso)
1 carbohydrate	1 tablespoon arrowroot starch dissolved in 2 to 3 tablespoons cold purified water
	Ground black pepper and/or minced parsley or chives to garnish
2 protein	2 ounces skim or part-skim mozzarella, Colby, cheddar, or soy cheese, sliced or cubed into 4 portions

Instructions

1. Add oil to a 1-quart saucepan. Heat to medium setting. Add onions. Stir and cook for about 3 to 4 minutes, until tender. Add zucchini and garlic. Stir and cook for

about 2 to 3 minutes. Add water, soy flour, and nutritional yeast, but do not stir. Cover and bring to boil. Reduce heat to low and simmer for about 15 minutes until vegetables are tender.

2. Transfer mixture to a blender. Add dill or nutmeg and miso, then cover and process until smooth. Return mixture to the saucepan. Warm over medium-low heat. Dissolve arrowroot in cold water, then add to soup. Simmer and stir until thick.

3. Remove from heat and serve warm, portioned into 4 soup bowls. Alternatively, chill soup, then serve as a cold starter before a meal. Garnish soup with parsley, chives, or black pepper. Serve cheese on the side.

Variations

Replace zucchini with equal amount of summer squash (yellow patty pan squash).

Replace miso with 1 teaspoon finely ground sea salt, but add the salt in Step 1 above. Then serve 2 cups of cherry tomatoes (to provide 1 carbohydrate block) with the soup and cheese.

Middle Eastern Antipasto

Servings: 4 Appetizers (1 block each)

Block size	Ingredients
2 carbohydrate	1/2 cup prepared hummus
1/2 carbohydrate	2 celery hearts, cut into long thin sticks
1 carbohydrate	2 large carrots, peeled and cut into sticks
1/2 carbohydrate	1 cup cherry tomatoes
4 fat	12 black olives
4 protein	4 ounces reduced-fat goat cheese or soy cheese

Instructions

1. Spoon hummus onto center of medium serving plate.

2. Arrange celery sticks, carrot sticks, tomatoes, olives, and cheese around hummus. Serve at room temperature.

Parboiled Vegetable Plate with Tofu Dip

Servings: 4 Appetizers (1 block each)

Block size	Ingredients
1/2 carbohydrate, 4 protein	3/4 pound regular tofu (not extra-firm)
	1 1/2 tablespoons umeboshi vinegar
	1 tablespoon brown rice vinegar or fresh lemon juice
	1 1/2 tablespoons Dijon or stone ground mustard
	Optional: 2 scallions, trimmed and minced
4 fat	1 1/3 teaspoons olive oil, or 12 black olives, chopped
	2 to 4 tablespoons purified water
	3 cups purified water
	1/2 teaspoon sea salt
1 carbohydrate	12 asparagus spears
1/2 carbohydrate	2 cups cauliflower, cut into bite-size florets
1 carbohydrate	1 large daikon (Japanese white radish), cut into sticks
1/2 carbohydrate	1 red or orange bell pepper, seeded, cut into long strips

Instructions

1. Boil or steam tofu for 4 minutes, then drain.

2. Crumble tofu into a blender or food processor. Add seasonings and olive oil. Blend until smooth and creamy. Add water a tablespoon or two at a time as needed to create a smooth texture like sour cream. Pour into 4 custard cups, cover, and chill for at least 3 hours to allow flavors to meld.

3. Meanwhile, bring 3 cups salted water to a boil in an uncovered 2-quart saucepan. Cook each type of vegetable separately but in the same boiling water, until crisp but tender. Cook about 2 to 4 minutes: more for asparagus and cauliflower, less for bell peppers.

4. Remove vegetables with a large skimmer basket and transfer to a colander. Run vegetables under cold water to stop the cooking and hold the color.

5. Place each dish of tofu dip on a large dinner plate. Arrange vegetables in concentric circles or mounds around the dish. Serve cold.

Vegetable Antipasto Plate

Servings: 4 Appetizers (1 block each)

Block size	Ingredients
2 carbohydrate	½ cup hummus
½ carbohydrate	4 celery hearts, cut into long thin sticks
1 carbohydrate	1 medium carrot, cut into sticks
½ carbohydrate	1 cup cherry tomatoes or low-acid gold "cherry" tomatoes
4 fat	12 almonds, chopped
4 protein	6 ounces smoked tofu, cut into a dozen long strips

Instructions

1. Divide hummus into four small mounds on appetizer plates.

2. Arrange vegetables, almonds, and tofu strips in concentric circles around the hummus.

3. Serve immediately or cover and chill.

Variation

Replace smoked tofu with 4 ounces of low-fat string cheese cut in strips.

Crudité Plate with Tofu Cream Cheese

Servings: 4 Appetizers (1 block each)

Block size	Ingredients
Block size	**Ingredients**
4 protein	³/₄ pound firm tofu
4 fat	2 teaspoons roasted sesame tahini
	2 tablespoons white, yellow, sweet, or mellow miso paste (NOT dark brown or red miso)
	1 tablespoon ume paste or 2 tablespoons ume/umeboshi vinegar
	3 tablespoons dried chives or ¹/₂ cup fresh chives, finely minced
	4 tablespoons purified water
	Optional: 2 to 3 cloves garlic, minced or pressed
	Optional: 6 sprigs of parsley, minced
¹/₂ carbohydrate	1 medium head of broccoli, cut into bite-size florets
¹/₂ carbohydrate	2 cups cauliflower, cut into bite-size florets
¹/₂ carbohydrate	1 orange bell pepper, seeded, cut in long, wide strips
¹/₂ carbohydrate	1 red or yellow bell pepper, seeded, cut in long, wide strips
	3 cups purified water
	¹/₂ teaspoon sea salt
1 carbohydrate	1 large tomato or 2 medium tomatoes, cut into wedges
1 carbohydrate	1 can artichoke hearts, drained

Instructions

1. Boil or steam tofu for about 3 minutes. Drain. Crumble tofu into a blender or food processor. Add tahini, miso, ume, and chives. Blend until smooth and creamy,

adding water a tablespoon at a time, only as needed to create a smooth texture like sour cream.

2. Pour into a bowl, cover, and chill at least 3 hours to allow flavors to meld.

3. Meanwhile, bring 3 cups salted water to a boil in an uncovered 2-quart saucepan. Cook each type of vegetable separately but in the same boiling water, until crisp but tender. Cook about 2 to 4 minutes: more for asparagus and cauliflower, less for bell peppers.

4. Remove vegetables with a large skimmer basket and transfer to a colander. Run vegetables under cold water to stop the cooking and hold the color.

5. Divide dip between 4 custard cups or ramekins and place each one on a large dinner plate. Arrange cold vegetables in concentric circles or mounds around the dish. Add tomato and artichoke hearts to each plate. Serve cold.

Modifying Your Favorite Recipes

Chapter 5 gave you more than 100 recipes for great Soy Zone meals. I realize, though, that you're probably not inclined to follow a recipe for every meal. How can you incorporate the Soy Zone into your everyday eating plan? That's precisely the point of this chapter.

I admit that I still enjoy lasagna occasionally—on a once- or twice-a-month basis. A recipe that my wife, Lynn, created uses six lasagna noodles instead of the traditional nine in a family-sized lasagna pan. This makes two layers instead of three. For the layers, she mixes together soy hamburger crumbles, a good tomato sauce filled with mushrooms and finely chopped vegetables, low-fat mozzarella cheese, and non-fat ricotta cheese made even tastier by a good infusion of pesto. (This recipe combines soy protein with dairy protein, but you could substitute the mozzarella cheese with soy cheese and the ricotta with silken tofu.)

I also realize that it's unrealistic to cook separate meals for you and your family. Families can be the biggest saboteurs when it comes to adopting healthful eating habits. And no parent wants to be a short-order cook. Without a doubt, the Soy Zone is the best eating plan for kids from a nutritional standpoint. Getting kids to try new foods, though, may not be a picnic unless they look like the foods they already eat. That's why I suggest you introduce soy products slowly, by using items such as soy sausage as a topping on their pizza, or soy hamburger crumbles in their favorite chili. If you're already making Zone meals, you can transform any of your favorite meals into Soy Zone meals by substituting the animal protein with a soy protein. This is not always as simple as it seems, since the density of protein in various soy products can vary dramatically. Here are some good rules for replacing animal protein in a Zone meal with various types of soy protein for women and men.

WOMEN

The typical Zone meal for a woman will usually contain 3 ounces of low-fat protein. This translates into approximately 20 grams of protein. Any one of the following soy products can replace 20 grams of protein:

$1^1/_2$ cups of boiled soybeans*

6 oz of extra-firm tofu

9 oz of firm tofu

12 oz of soft tofu

15 oz of silken tofu

12 oz of tempeh*

1 cup of soy hamburger crumbles

$1^1/_2$ soy hamburger patties

3 soy sausage patties

3 soy hot dogs

$4^1/_2$ slices of soy deli meat substitute

3 tablespoons of textured soy protein

20 grams of soy protein powder

3 oz of soy cheese

24 oz of soy yogurt*

18 oz of soy milk*

*Contains extra carbohydrate, so read the label carefully.

MEN

The typical Zone meal for a man will usually contain 4 ounces of low-fat protein. This translates into approximately 30 grams of protein. Any one of the following soy products can replace 30 grams of protein:

2 cups of boiled soybeans*

8 oz of extra-firm tofu

12 oz of firm tofu

16 oz of soft tofu

20 oz of silken tofu

20 oz of tempeh*

1¹/₃ cups of soy hamburger crumbles

2 soy hamburger patties

4 soy sausage patties

4 soy hot dogs

6 slices of soy deli meat substitute

4 tablespoons of textured vegetable protein

20 grams of soy protein powder

4 oz of soy cheese

32 oz of soy yogurt*

24 oz of soy milk*

*Contains extra carbohydrate, so read the label carefully.

Getting Your Body Used to Soy Products

Although beans usually cause few problems for people who eat them often, they may cause some discomfort when you first start adding them to your diet. The same holds true for soybeans and soy products rich in fiber. For the first several weeks, your digestive system may have trouble breaking down all the oligosaccharides (complex sugars not readily absorbed) in beans, so bacteria in the large intestines ferment these sugars and produce gas as a by-product. As a result, you may feel bloated, or you may experience flatulence, excessive belching, or stomach pains if you suddenly go on a high-soy diet. Over time, your body will get used to the soy in your diet, and you'll probably find that your symptoms go away on their own. Until then, you can try these strategies:

- Stick mainly with tofu, tempeh, and soy milk, which are more easily digested, even by people who have trouble with whole beans.

- Use soy meat substitutes in which most of the fiber has been removed.

- Eat very small portions of any soy products that give you trouble. Gradually increase your portion size over several months.

- Be sure that soybeans are thoroughly cooked.

- Try a product such as Beano to break down the indigestible sugars before they get to the bacteria in your large intestine.

- Fortify meals with soy protein isolates, which are almost pure protein.

- Whole soybeans, textured soy protein, soy flour, and soy grits are high in fiber, so be sure to drink plenty of liquids to aid digestion.

SOY ZONE MEALS FOR KIDS

There is a soy revolution going on as far as children are concerned. The U.S. government has started a push to get soy foods included in school lunches. Worried about the high amounts of saturated fat in children's meals, the U.S. Department of Agriculture is now encouraging schools and day care centers to serve tofu, veggie burgers, and other soy products as meat substitutes in federally subsidized lunches. Of course, getting kids to eat soy foods can be the biggest obstacle. I can only emphasize again that any soy protein product had better look like and taste like hamburgers, salami, and hot dogs before kids are going to embrace them. You may find that you'll have more success getting your kids to eat soy meals that you prepare at home than the often tasteless meals they get in the school cafeteria. Here are some tips for getting your kids into the Soy Zone.

1. **Start them early—the younger, the better.** You'll be doing your kids a great favor by raising them on more soy foods. Younger children tend to be more adaptable than older children and are more willing to try something new. However, with young children, be aware that some may have allergies to soy protein (see below).

2. **Enter soy in disguise.** Rather than serving a piece of tofu to your family, disguise soy in their favorite foods. Make them a fruit smoothie made with soy protein powder or a meat loaf made with half extra-lean ground beef and half soy hamburger crumbles. Also, try making a dip for their carrot sticks from tofu and packaged dry onion soup.

3. **Older children may not want to try new foods, so be subtle and go slowly.** Substitute soy flour for some of the flour in their favorite muffins. Use soy milk in cooking and baking, and keep their foods looking familiar. You don't even need to tell your family that they're eating soy. Let them try it before you tell them the dish has a new ingredient.

4. **Don't pressure them to eat soy.** As most parents know very well, pressuring children to do something can make them go in the exact

opposite direction. Even if your children are reluctant to eat soy, keep serving them small portions, without comment. Don't require them to eat half or even take a bite. Just let them see you eating it. Persistence usually pays off, and most children will try a new food eventually.

5. **Acknowledge the fact that soy foods taste a little different.** Don't pretend that a soy burger tastes exactly like a hamburger. Your children will think you're trying to pull one over on them. Let them tell you what they think of the taste, or tell them what you think of the food. For instance, you can introduce soy milk as "fancy milk for a special treat." Plan to use lots of condiments like catsup, mustard, or relish to alter the taste to what they're accustomed to. Also, don't be afraid of using a little extra olive oil or sprinkling of nuts to improve a food's taste. After a while, your kids will be used to seeing soy foods in the house and not think of them as different or strange.

6. **Introduce a variety of soy foods, and let your kids decide what they like.** With all the choices out there, let your kids plan their own soy menus with the foods they like. Maybe they prefer a particular brand of soy burger, or they prefer soy sausage links to soy hot dogs. As with any food, your kids will only eat what they like.

7. **Remember to serve your kids a meal that's balanced in terms of protein and carbohydrate.** It makes little hormonal sense to have them consume a little more soy protein if they are still eating massive amounts of carbohydrates.

How much protein do children need?

Modifying your favorite kids' meals with soy protein is easier than you think, especially with the development of soy protein meat substitutes. However, you may be wondering how much protein your child needs and what percentage should be soy protein.

For kids ages 2 to 12, I usually recommend that each meal contain at least 10 grams of protein. If they are very active, you may want to increase their protein intake to 15 grams per meal. For children under age 2, make sure you add extra fat to their diet (in the form of infant formulas and whole-milk dairy products), since they require a greater intake of this nutrient to spur brain growth and development. A 10-gram serving of protein is equivalent to $1^1/_2$ ounces of low-fat protein. You can find this amount of protein in these servings of soy protein products:

$^3/_4$ cup of boiled soybeans*

3 oz of extra-firm tofu

$4^1/_2$ oz of firm tofu

6 oz of soft tofu

$7^1/_2$ oz of silken tofu

6 oz of tempeh*

$^1/_2$ cup of soy hamburger crumbles

$^3/_4$ soy hamburger patty

$1^1/_2$ soy sausage patties

$1^1/_2$ soy hot dogs

2 slices of soy deli meat substitute

$1^1/_2$ tablespoons of textured soy protein

10 grams of soy protein powder

$1^1/_2$ oz of soy cheese

12 oz of soy yogurt*

9 oz of soy milk*

*Contains extra carbohydrate, so read the label carefully.

If children eat three Zone meals per day, each containing about 10 grams of protein, and two Zone snacks, each containing about 7 grams of protein, their total protein intake should be approximately 45 grams of protein per day. As with adults, I usually recommend that about half of that protein (about 22 grams per day) should be soy protein. This means that your kids can either eat two meals each day completely composed of soy protein, or alternatively have one meal composed of soy protein in addition to two Zone snacks composed of soy protein. This allows you to maintain a variety of other protein sources for your children in addition to soy protein.

TEENAGERS

After puberty, I treat teenagers as adults relative to the their protein requirements. They should follow the guidelines listed above for substituting soy protein for the protein in their favorite meals. Again, like adults, they will achieve maximum health benefits by ensuring that the rest of the meal is balanced with respect to protein and carbohydrates.

Soy Food Allergies

Just as some children are allergic to cow's milk, some are allergic to soy protein. The incidence of cow's milk allergy ranges from 0.3 to 7.5 percent among infants. Allergy to soy is seen in 0.5 percent of infants. By age 2, the majority of children outgrow their allergies to soy, and soy allergies are uncommon in adults. Soy protein-based formulas are an excellent alternative for infants who are allergic to dairy-based formulas. By the same token, dairy formulas are an excellent alternative for infants who are allergic to soy. Various studies, however, have found that soy formulas hold no advantage over cow's milk formula in the prevention of childhood allergies. Of course, breastfeeding remains the ideal infant formula.

Soy allergies can manifest themselves through an array of symptoms similar to those of other food allergies. If your child develops any of the following symptoms after eating soy products, you should consult your pediatrician to see if the symptoms are related to a soy allergy.

- diarrhea

- vomiting

- sneezing

- watery eyes

- nasal congestion

- skin rash, itchy skin swellings, or hives

- stomach upset

- wheezing or trouble breathing

- swelling in the tongue or throat

Allergies can be diagnosed from your child's medical history, symptoms, skin patch tests (where a tiny amount of soy is rubbed on the skin to see the reaction), or a blood test to identify the allergen. Children who are allergic to soy can benefit from the regular Zone Diet, as it will decrease the overactive immune response to the soy protein. If you wish to raise your children as vegans and they have allergies to soy protein, you can substitute rice protein powder.

USING SOY FOOD INGREDIENTS TO SUBSTITUTE IN YOUR FAVORITE MEALS

This list shows easy ways to substitute soy food ingredients in dips, salad dressings, soups, stews, shakes, entrees, sandwiches, and desserts. While the reductions may seem small, over time they add up to better health when incorporated into a well-balanced diet.

Guide to Modifying Recipes: One-to-One Substitutions

- 1 cup milk = 1 cup fortified soy milk

- 1 cup fruit yogurt = 1 cup soft silken tofu + $^1/_2$ cup of fruit of your choice, blended together

- 1 egg = 1 tablespoon soy flour + 1 tablespoon water

- 1 egg = 1 to 2-inch square of tofu

- 1 cup ricotta cheese = 1 cup firm tofu, mashed

- 2 tablespoons flour = 1 tablespoon soy flour

- Replace $^1/_2$ of the flour in self-rising baked goods with soy flour

- Replace $^1/_3$ cup of the flour in quick breads with soy flour

- 1 ounce ground beef = $^1/_3$ cup soy hamburger crumbles

- 1 ounce cheddar cheese = 1 ounce soy cheese

Fine-Tuning the Soy Zone Diet

The point of the Soy Zone is to achieve one specific goal: to maintain steady insulin levels within the Zone. Most of us can do this by following the eyeball method that I outlined in Chapter 2. Some of us, though, need to make adjustments to calculate the precise amount of protein our own bodies need.

For example, if you engage in an intense weight-training regimen or exercise vigorously, you're going to need to eat more protein (and also carbohydrates) than the average man or woman. You may also require more protein if you're obese—more than 30 percent above your ideal body weight.

If you've eaten a meal that has put you in the Zone, you should feel this way for the next 4 to 6 hours after eating:

- Lack of hunger.

- Lack of carbohydrate cravings.

- Good mental focus and clarity.

- Good physical performance.

HOW TO TELL IF YOU NEED FINE-TUNING

How can you tell if you need to make some adjustments in your Soy Zone eating plan? Here's a simple test: Eat a meal and note the time.

Four hours later, ask yourself two questions: (1) Are you hungry? and (2) Do you have a good mental focus? If you're not hungry and you have a good mental focus, then you know your last meal put you in the Zone.

On the other hand, if four hours after a meal you are hungry and you have poor mental focus, you probably ate too many carbohydrates relative to protein. As I already discussed, eating a meal that contains primarily carbohydrates causes your insulin levels to shoot way up, which then causes your blood sugar levels to plunge way down. So three or four hours after eating, say, a big pasta meal for lunch, you're left feeling exhausted and mentally drained. In essence, you're paying the hormonal price of increased insulin production. You need to take note of how you're feeling after every meal. If you feel depleted a few hours after eating, keep your protein constant but decrease the amount of carbohydrate the next time you eat that same meal.

If, on the other hand, you're hungry three or four hours after eating, but you have good mental focus, then you've had too few carbohydrates relative to the amount of protein. What you've done is pushed your insulin levels too low. The solution? Add more low-density carbohydrates the next time you eat that same meal, while keeping your protein intake the same.

IT'S ALL IN THE MATH

So far, I've discussed getting into the Zone by giving you some simple rules: Eyeball your portions; divide your plate into sections; eat a piece of soy protein no larger than the size and thickness of your palm. The Zone, however, is based upon mathematical principles in which stable insulin levels are achieved by eating a specific ratio of protein to carbohydrates. In fact, there is a bell-shaped curve of protein-to-carbohydrates ratios that will keep you in the Zone, as shown in the figure on page 195.

If you consume more than twice as many carbohydrates as protein at a meal (a protein-to-carbohydrate ratio of less than 0.5), then you will be producing too much insulin. On the other hand, if you are eating more protein than carbohydrate at a meal (a protein-to-carbohydrate ratio greater than 1.0), you will be producing too much of the

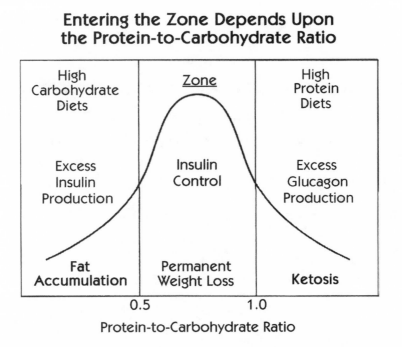

Entering the Zone Depends Upon the Protein-to-Carbohydrate Ratio

Protein-to-Carbohydrate Ratio

hormone glucagon. Reaching the Zone is like being Goldilocks on a quest for the right bowl of porridge—not too hot (too much insulin), not too cold (too much glucagon), but just right (in the Zone).

If you suspect that you're not getting the maximum benefits of the Soy Zone Diet, you can use this chapter to do some fine-tuning. The first step of that process is to determine your exact protein requirements, and that begins by determining your percentage of body fat.

Your goal on the Soy Zone Diet is to lose excess body fat while maintaining your muscle or lean body mass. This is why adequate protein intake is essential—to maintain or even increase your lean body mass. On the other hand, your fat mass doesn't require any incoming protein whatsoever. In fact, you can gain as much fat as you want (like you'd really want to!) just by eating excess carbohydrates. For this reason, your individualized protein prescription will be based only on the pounds that make up your lean body mass—which is your total weight minus your pounds of fat. You can figure out how many pounds of fat you have by determining your body fat percentage. You can easily calculate your body fat percentage by following the instructions in Appendix C.

YOUR INDIVIDUALIZED PROTEIN PRESCRIPTION

Your personalized protein prescription is based on your lean body mass and your physical activity level. To calculate your lean body mass, you must first calculate how many pounds of fat you have and then subtract this from your total weight. Here is the equation:

Your total body weight x Your body fat percentage =
Your fat mass (total pounds of body fat)

Let's say you're a typical male who weighs 180 pounds and has 20 percent body fat. Your total fat mass would then be:

180 lbs X 0.20 = 36 pounds

This means you have 36 pounds of pure fat on your body. Since each pound of fat contains 3,500 calories of energy, you have the equivalent of

36 lbs fat x 3,500 calories/lb fat = 126,000 calories in storage

That's a lot of stored energy, in fact enough to run more than 50 marathons back-to-back, if only you could access it. Unfortunately, if you have high levels of insulin, you can't access this virtually unlimited amount of stored energy because excess insulin blocks its release.

Lean body mass is simply your total weight minus your total fat. In the example above, this 180-pound individual would have

180 pounds total weight - 36 pounds of fat =
144 pounds of lean body mass

It's these 144 pounds of lean body mass that require incoming dietary protein for maintenance.

In addition to your lean body mass, you need to factor in the amount of exercise you get on a regular basis. Do you lie on the couch and watch TV when you're not spending your time staring at a computer screen? Or do you work out twice a day? The greater the level of your physical activity, the greater the amount of protein you need to maintain your lean body mass. Remember that exercise causes the breakdown of muscle tissue and consequently more dietary protein is required to repair the existing muscle cells as well as to build new muscle tissue. Choose your level of activity from the table below and plug the coinciding number into the equation below to determine your protein prescription.

Physical Activity and Protein Requirements	
Level of Activity	**Grams of Protein/Pound of Lean Body Mass**
Sedentary	0.5
Light activity (i.e. walking)	0.6
Moderate (1.5 hours per week)	0.7
Active (1.5 to 2.5 hours per week)	0.8
Very Active (greater than 2.5 hours per week)	0.9
Elite Athlete	1.0

The equation to determine your protein prescription is the following:

Lean body mass X Grams of protein/pound of lean body mass = Protein prescription

Using the example above, let's assume that you're a 180-pound male with 20 percent body fat who works out for 30 minutes three times a week—a total of 1.5 hours of physical activity. Remember, we already calculated your lean body mass to be 144 pounds. Your protein prescription would be:

144 lbs X 0.7 grams of protein = 100 grams of protein

So in this example, you should consume a total of 100 grams of protein throughout the day. That's why I recommend *no more* than 30 grams of protein at each meal for the average American male. Three Soy Zone meals plus two Soy Zone snacks (at 7 grams of protein) would provide about 100 grams of protein per day.

Let's do the same calculation for a typical female who weighs 150 pounds and has 30 percent body fat. First let's calculate her total fat mass:

$$150 \text{ lbs} \times 0.30 = 45 \text{ pounds of fat}$$

Now we can calculate the lean body mass of this person.

$$150 \text{ lbs} - 45 \text{ lbs of fat} = 105 \text{ lbs of lean body mass}$$

If this female exercises three times a week for 30 minutes, then her activity factor would be 0.7 grams/lb. lean body mass. Finally, we can calculate her protein requirements.

$$105 \text{ lbs of lean body mass} \times 0.7 \text{ g/lb LBM} = 74 \text{ grams}$$

So if this female is eating *no more* than 20 grams of protein at a meal three times per day and having two Zone snacks with 7 grams each, by the end of the day she will have consumed about 75 grams of protein. So now you can understand the math behind my general recommendations for how much protein you need.

Here's a quick summary of the steps for determining your protein prescription:

1. Determine your body fat percentage from Appendix C

2. Calculate your total fat mass

3. Calculate your lean body mass

4. Determine your level of physical activity

5. Calculate the grams of protein you should eat on a daily basis

After calculating your protein prescription, you may discover that you need to eat less protein than the 75 grams recommended for women or the 100 grams recommended for men. Regardless of your calculations, I strongly recommend that you stick with no less than 75 grams of protein each day. This would mean eating about 20 grams of protein per Soy Zone meal and two Soy Zone snacks containing about 7 grams of protein each.

After years of clinical studies with Type 2 diabetics, I have found that this *minimum* recommendation of 75 grams of protein per day works exceptionally well for both diabetics and the general population. Even at 75 grams of protein per day, you are still eating less protein than the Okinawans.

Keep in mind that the Soy Zone Diet is not a "diet" in the traditional sense. Diets are usually thought of as quick fixes that take off weight temporarily, until you return to your old eating habits, which originally caused the weight gain in the first place. The Soy Zone Diet is a lifelong food management program based on balance and moderation for better insulin control. Think of being in the Zone as having a hormonal checkbook. Like your regular checkbook, you don't have to balance it to the penny to make it work. You only want to make sure that there is enough money in the account so that the next check you write doesn't bounce. The Zone is similar. You want the best possible balance of protein and carbohydrate at each meal so that the hormonal checks you are going to write don't bounce during the next four to six hours.

At this point, you have two options: The first option is to just continue to use the eyeball method and try some of the recipes for the Soy Zone meals in Chapter 5, which provide approximately 30 grams of protein per serving. Using the recipes is the easier of the two options because it requires the least amount of effort and calculations.

Your second option is to fine-tune the Soy Zone Diet using your personal protein prescription. This requires a little more effort on your part, but it will allow you to have more control over your insulin levels and optimize your own unique biochemistry. If you choose this option, you can use one of two food accounting methods that I have developed. One is called the "1–2–3" method, and the other is the Zone Food Block method. Both are described below.

THE "1-2-3" METHOD

The "1-2-3" method means that for every *one* gram of fat you eat, you should have *two* grams of protein and *three* grams of carbohydrate. Therefore a typical Soy Zone meal for a female (who needs about 20 grams of protein per meal) would contain 10 grams of fat, 20 grams of protein, and 30 grams of carbohydrate. For the average male (who needs about 30 grams of protein per meal), a Soy Zone meal would contain 15 grams of fat, 30 grams of protein, and 45 grams of carbohydrate. A typical Zone snack would have 3 grams of fat, 6 grams of protein, and 9 grams of carbohydrate.

THE ZONE FOOD BLOCK METHOD

I realize that you may have a hard time keeping track of the number of protein, carbohydrate, and fat grams at every meal. So to simplify this accounting system, I developed another method known as Zone Food Blocks. This is a food exchange system that allows you to get the right balance of protein, carbohydrate, and fat at every meal and snack. One Protein Block contains 7 grams of protein; one Carbohydrate Block contains 9 grams; one Fat Block contains 3 grams. All the recipes in Chapter 5 are broken down into Zone Food Blocks.

For all Soy Zone meals, meal preparation starts with the amount of protein you need. For the typical American female, that will be about 20 grams per meal. That number can be converted into Zone Food Blocks as follows:

20 grams protein ÷ 7 grams protein/Zone Food Block = approximately 3 Zone Blocks

For the average American male, who needs about 30 grams of protein per meal, the calculation of Zone Food Blocks is the same.

30 grams protein ÷ 7 grams protein/Zone Food Block = approximately 4 Zone Blocks

Since the Zone is all about balancing the foods you eat, you can probably guess how many carbohydrate and fat blocks you need if you have three protein blocks. That's right—three of each. If you have four protein blocks, you would have four fat blocks and four carbohydrate blocks. At each snack, you should have one block each of protein, carbohydrate, and fat.

With the Zone Food Block system, the mathematics of preparing a Soy Zone meal are simple: for every Zone Protein Block you consume, add one Zone Carbohydrate Block and one Zone Fat Block. Stop adding the Zone Blocks when you reach your total required number for that meal. In Appendix D, you'll find a table of foods broken down into Zone Food Blocks. Although the Zone Food Block method takes a little time to get used to, you'll find it much easier to use, especially when it comes to fine-tuning your Soy Zone Diet.

The Zone Food Block method comes in handy if you feel as if your last meal didn't get you into the Zone. If you're fatigued and mentally drained after having a meal, have that exact same meal in a few days but keep the protein constant while *decreasing* the carbohydrate content of that meal by one Zone block (or by 10 grams if you are using the "1–2–3" method). By the same token, if you are hungry and have good mental focus after a meal, you should again try having the exact same meal, but this time *increase* the carbohydrate content of that meal by one Zone Carbohydrate Block or 10 grams.

WHAT IT TAKES TO MASTER THE ZONE

Just as you can achieve different-colored belts based on commitment and skill in the martial arts, so can you achieve different levels on the way to becoming a Zone Master. The difference is that in the Zone you can start right at Level 3, or you can work your way from Level 1 to Level 3—stopping at the level that you feel comfortable doing on a consistent basis. Here's all the information you need to master the Zone, starting with the easiest to the most advanced level.

Level 1: Follow the Commonsense Rules of Eating Like Your Grandmother Taught You

1. Eat more fruits and vegetables, and less pasta, breads, grains, and starches.

2. Eat small amounts of low-fat protein (but no larger nor thicker than the palm of your hand) at every meal.

3. Eat smaller, more frequent meals that contain fewer calories.

Level 2: Start to Pay Attention

1. Follow the eyeball method at every meal by filling your plate with two-thirds low-density carbohydrates and one-third protein.

2. Add some monounsaturated fat at every meal.

3. Take long-chain Omega-3 fatty acid and vitamin E supplements every day.

Level 3: Begin Thinking Hormonally

1. Determine how much protein you need each day and spread it over three meals and two snacks.

2. Try to keep your intake of pasta, breads, grains, and starches to a minimum, eating primarily vegetables and fruits.

3. Never let more than five hours go by without eating a Zone meal or snack.

4. Always eat a Zone breakfast within one hour after waking.

5. Always have a small Zone snack before you go to bed.

Even at the most advanced level, the Soy Zone Diet doesn't require a great deal of effort. You just need to remember that if you want to feel balanced and have your body's systems finely tuned, then you'll need to eat the right combination of foods. You also need to remember that you're the one in control and that you're the one who decides whether you abuse the drug called food or use it as a medicine to heal your body and help you live a longer life.

Your Longevity Report Card: The Tests You Want to Pass

8

Do you want to know how well you're doing in reaching your goal of greater longevity? Of course you do. If you only had a report card that could accurately tell you how close you are to reaching your goal of a longer and healthier life. Actually, such a report card exists, based on two distinct types of tests. The first type of tests you can do yourself, based on your body fat percentage and your strength. The second series of tests involves blood work, which your doctor needs to order.

Being on the Soy Zone entails more than just eating the right kinds of foods in the right balance. You can't neglect exercise because it's a vital part of any healthy lifestyle. Why do you need to worry about physical activity if you're eating nutritiously? Once again, it all comes back to insulin. In order to maximize the control over your insulin levels, you need to eat a Zone diet and also get regular physical activity. I believe that eating in the Zone takes you about 80 percent there and that exercise takes you the rest of the way.

Exercise won't improve your insulin levels if you're eating tons of carbohydrates. It will, though, amplify the benefits of the Soy Zone Diet. The point of this chapter is to assess where you're at right now. How physically fit are you? What is your body fat percentage? How are your insulin levels and lipid levels? These tests will give you a clear indication of how you're doing and where you should aim to improve. The best part about them is that *you will see an improvement in the results if you follow the Soy Zone*. Thus, you can take them periodically to monitor your efforts on the Soy Zone.

These tests will serve as your report card to tell you how close you are to reaching your goal of a longer and healthier life.

TESTS YOU CAN DO YOURSELF

Certain physical markers can give you some indication as to whether you have healthy or dangerous levels of insulin. One factor is your body fat distribution. Do you tend to have more fat on your stomach (apple shape)? Or more on your hips and thighs (pear shape)? If you're an apple shape, you're at much higher risk of having unhealthy insulin levels and of developing heart disease and diabetes.

1. Measuring Your Body Fat Percentage:

Your percentage of body fat is an even more precise indicator than body fat distribution about whether you have unhealthy insulin levels. To determine your percentage of body fat, follow the directions in Appendix C.

Write in your body fat percentage: _____

If you're a woman, you should aim for a body fat percentage of 22 percent. If you're a man, your goal should be approximately 15 percent. **If your percentage of body fat is more than 25 percent for males and more than 33 percent for females, you are making too much insulin.** Unfortunately, more than half the adult population in America exceeds these percentages of body fat, which means that the majority of us have unhealthy insulin levels. This is the largest health epidemic in our nation today, yet it goes largely untreated.

Your body weight doesn't always serve as the best parameter for your health. If you add muscle mass, you can actually gain weight, while decreasing your body fat percentage. Measuring your body fat percentage will give you a far more reliable predictor of your future health. In fact, even thin people can have a decreased longevity if they don't have enough muscle (lean body mass). This is why there are some thin people walking around who have elevated insulin levels.

2. Measuring Your Body Strength:

Make no mistake about it: The quality of your life is strongly dependent on your upper-body and lower-body strength. Simple tasks like walking up stairs or carrying the groceries in from the car become much more difficult as you lose strength. One of the problems of traditional grain-based vegetarian diets is that they often lack adequate protein to maintain your muscle mass.

You can easily test both your upper-body and lower-body strength by doing some simple exercises. For the upper-body test you can do push-ups (different types for men and women). Men can do the classic push-up with the arms in a direct line with the shoulders. Women can do modified push-ups with their knees on the floor, but again with the arms in a direct line from the shoulders. Always make sure that your back is not sagging (pull your abdominal muscles in) and that you are touching the floor with your chest and not your chin. Remember, no one is watching you, but you still want an honest assessment of your current strength. The table below shows how upper-body strength is measured for both males and females.

Tests for Upper-Body Strength

A. Push-Ups for Men

Age:	20–29	30–39	40–49	50–59	>60
Fitness Level					
Excellent	>55	>45	>40	>35	>30
Good	45–54	35–44	30–39	25–34	20–29
Average	35–44	25–34	20–29	15–24	10–19
Fair	20–34	15–24	12–19	8–14	5–9
Low	0–19	0–14	0–11	0–7	0–4

B. Modified Knee Push-Ups for Women

Age:	20–29	30–39	40–49	50–59	>60
Fitness Level					
Excellent	>49	>40	>35	>30	>20
Good	34–48	25–39	20–34	15–29	5–19
Average	17–33	12–24	8–19	6–14	3–4
Fair	6–16	4–11	3–7	2–5	1–2
Low	0–5	0–3	0–2	0–1	0

Write down how many push-ups you can do: _____

My prescription for upper body strength: Do as many push-ups as you can three times a week. It's most important to maintain good form. Do fewer repetitions, rather than give up your form. Work your way up to two sets of 30 or more.

Lower-body strength can be measured by performing leg squats using weights. To do this test, use a chair of standard height (approximately 18 to 20 inches) without arms. If you're a man, hold 15-pound dumbbells in each hand (a total of 30 pounds). If you're a woman, hold 5-pound dumbbells in each hand (a total of 10 pounds). Keeping your legs as wide as your hips, bend your knees and lower yourself until you touch the seat of the chair and then return to your starting position. Do as many repetitions as you can while maintaining good form. Then check out how you rate in lower-body strength as shown in the following table.

Tests for Lower-Body Strength

A. 30-Pound Squats for Men

Age:	20–29	30–39	40–49	50–59	>60
Fitness Level					
Excellent	>55	>45	>40	>35	>30
Good	45–54	35–44	30–39	25–34	20–29
Average	35–44	25–34	20–29	15–24	10–19
Fair	20–34	15–24	12–19	8–14	5–9
Low	0–19	0–14	0–11	0–7	0–4

B. 10-Pound Squats for Women

Age:	20–29	30–39	40–49	50–59	>60
Fitness Level					
Excellent	>49	>40	>35	>30	>20
Good	34–48	25–39	20–34	15–29	5–19
Average	17–33	12–24	8–19	6–14	3–4
Fair	6–16	4–11	3–7	2–5	1–2
Low	0–5	0–3	0–2	0–1	0

Write down how many squats you can do: _____

My prescription for improving your lower body strength: Do as many squats as you can (without using any weights), three times a week. Work your way up to two sets of 40 squats at a time three times a week.

For both upper- and lower-body strength, your goal is to meet, if not exceed, the "good" fitness level at any age.

The importance of maintaining your body strength is that it will determine how well you function later in life. It can also improve your energy levels now by making everyday tasks a lot easier. Your strength indicates whether or not you are getting enough protein in your diet. However, without a consistent exercise program, all the protein in the world will not maintain, let alone increase, your lean muscle mass.

My prescription for aerobic exercise: Your exercise program should also consist of aerobic or steady exercise. One of the best ways to condition your heart is by walking. I recommend walking 30 minutes every day, either all at once or in three 10-minute spurts throughout the day. The scientific data are quite clear that exercising 30 to 40 minutes a day has a dramatic impact on the reduction of heart disease, Type 2 diabetes, and cancer. It's not hard; you just have get into the routine and make it an everyday part of your life, like brushing your teeth.

TESTS THAT YOUR DOCTOR *MUST* ADMINISTER

Your blood does not have a political agenda. It tells you whether you've been good to your body or bad. More important, it will tell you what dietary changes you need to make to increase the likelihood of living longer. The blood tests I'm recommending are the standard ones used to monitor the millions of Type 2 diabetics in this country whose condition is caused by an overproduction of insulin. If your goal is optimal health, then these are the two blood tests you want to pass every time you take them:

1. Fasting insulin

2. Fasting triglyceride-to-HDL cholesterol ratio

Of the two tests, fasting insulin is the most important because it tells you how well you are maintaining that hormone within the Zone. *This single blood test is the best predictor of whether you will develop heart disease.* Unfortunately, this test is rarely done unless your doctor suspects that you have diabetes. The onus is on you to make sure your physician does a fasting insulin blood test at your next checkup. Lipid blood tests are much more common, although many doctors perform blood tests to measure your total cholesterol without giving information on the components of cholesterol (such as HDL levels) or triglyceride levels. Make sure you have a fasting blood test and get a breakdown of your total lipids that includes triglyceride levels (which usually rise with insulin levels) and your HDL (the "good" cholesterol). Then calculate your triglyceride-to-HDL ratio. This ratio is an indirect marker for insulin. The greater your triglycerides and the lower your HDL levels (the higher the ratio), the greater your risk of having a heart attack. The passing grades for these blood tests are shown in the table below.

Passing Grades for Longevity Based on Blood Tests			
Test	Ideal	Good	Fail
Insulin (μU/ml)	5	less than 10	more than 15
TG/HDL	less than 1	less than 2	more than 4

This is my scientific definition of the Zone: Maintaining your fasting insulin levels between 5 μU/ml and 10 μU/ml. It takes all of the politics out of nutrition, and makes nutrition a more clinical science, as it should be.

Write down your fasting insulin level: _____

Write down your fasting TG/HDL ratio: _____

YOUR LONGEVITY REPORT CARD

Filling out your overall longevity report card is pretty simple. Just measure your percentage of body fat and your strength at least once a month in your own home. Every six months, have your doctor run a blood test of your fasting insulin levels and your fasting cholesterol levels. These tests will tell you how well you are doing in your quest for a longer and healthier life. The following table shows you what a good report card looks like at any age.

Straight "A" Longevity Report Card	
Percent Body Fat	less than 15 percent (men)
	less than 22 percent (women)
Upper Body Strength	Rating equal, if not greater, than good
Lower Body Strength	Rating equal, if not greater, than good
Fasting Insulin	less than 10 µU/ml
TG/HDL Ratio	less than 2

These tests don't lie. If you haven't been following good nutritional habits, these tests will tell you. If you're consuming a traditional grain-based vegetarian diet (or any diet for that matter) and meet all of the above criteria, then don't change your diet. It's obviously working for you. If your test grades are disappointing, though, plan to make some changes in your diet and lifestyle. This means doing more strength-training exercises and getting into a cardiovascular routine that you can follow every day. It also means that you have to increase your efforts to follow the Soy Zone Diet.

Insulin: Your Body's Dr. Jekyll and Mr. Hyde

9

Now that you have begun to follow the rules of the Soy Zone Diet or have sampled some Soy Zone meals, you might be wondering why you're beginning to feel so good so quickly. Your improved mental focus, increased energy, and change in body composition have been effortlessly achieved without hunger, deprivation, or fatigue. These seemingly magical changes are simply a consequence of learning how to control the most powerful drug in the world: food.

As I stated earlier, the concept of treating food as if it were a drug began some 2,500 years ago, when Hippocrates said, "Let food be your medicine, and let medicine be your food." As we enter the 21st century, we can now update his wisdom by treating food as a medicine in order to keep insulin within the Zone. To understand the science behind the Soy Zone more fully, you first have to understand what hormones are and why insulin is the central character in this dietary drama.

INSULIN'S DUAL PERSONALITY

Imagine hormones as biological messengers that transmit information almost instantaneously to distant parts of your body. Since your body has some 60 trillion cells from your head to your toes, you can imagine how complex these interactions must be to maintain biological information flow. Among the hundreds of hormones discovered, insulin is probably the most widely studied because it is a storage hormone that tells the body to store incoming nutrients necessary for survival. Without an adequate supply of insulin, you would not be able to live.

When you have too much insulin, however, it actually begins to disrupt the flow of biological communication, which can cause your cells to go haywire. This can give rise to a host of life-threatening diseases, such as heart disease, adult-onset diabetes, and cancer.

Because of its dual personality, I consider insulin to be the Jekyll-and-Hyde hormone. Just like the heroic Dr. Jekyll inadvertently turned himself into the evil Mr. Hyde, insulin can either sustain your life or destroy it. When maintained at adequate levels and kept under control, insulin acts like the fearless Dr. Jekyll, selflessly delivering nutrients to cells in the body. This is why eating an adequate amount of carbohydrates is important: They are the primary stimulators of insulin secretion. Without adequate levels of insulin, your cells would starve to death.

Eating too many carbohydrates, however, can cause excess insulin secretion, which turns this otherwise heroic hormone into a raging monster, like the evil Mr. Hyde. Consuming too many calories at any one meal can also usher in the appearance of Mr. Hyde. Traditional grain-based vegetarian diets (as well as the standard American diet) can unleash Mr. Hyde because these diets are very rich in high-density carbohydrates, which promote insulin secretion.

Why do excess levels of insulin have such a negative impact on our health? Excess insulin disrupts the fidelity of your hormonal information systems, so that cells aren't able to transmit and receive messages at peak efficiency. It's like attempting a phone conversation with constant background noise over the wires. Excess insulin makes cellular communication difficult if not downright impossible. Instead of acting like well-oiled machines, your cells get a garbled message and may start dividing too rapidly or begin producing too much or not enough of a particular substance. These cellular malfunctions that excess insulin causes can lead to many of the diseases associated with aging, such as obesity, heart disease, cancer, or adult-onset (Type 2) diabetes.

WHAT WORKS AND WHAT DOESN'T

If you have excess levels of insulin, the best drug for reducing your levels is a completely natural one: food. Yes, the very same substance that caused your insulin levels to soar in the first place can also help your levels return to normal. The Soy Zone Diet can help you achieve just that: help you rein in your insulin levels and transform them back from Mr. Hyde into Dr. Jekyll. Thus, the hormonal key to a longer life is keeping insulin within the Zone: not too high, not too low. As I discussed in the last chapter, the Zone is a concrete measurement of your insulin. Your blood can show whether you're in the Zone—defined as a fasting insulin level of between 5 $\mu U/ml$ and 10 $\mu U/ml$.

About 75 percent of Americans have a genetic predisposition to make excess insulin when they consume too many carbohydrates. Unfortunately, about one-third of this group (about 25 percent of all Americans) have an extremely elevated insulin response to carbohydrates and thus are at very high risk for the development of heart disease and adult-onset diabetes. The other two-thirds of the group (about 50 percent of Americans) have just a slightly lower insulin response to carbohydrates and are at elevated risk for developing diabetes and heart disease if they consume excess carbohydrates. Both of these groups may suffer severe health consequences if they follow the grain-based diet recommended by the U.S. government. Just 25 percent of Americans have a very low insulin response, regardless of the amount of carbohydrates they eat; they are the lucky ones, genetically speaking. They will do well on any high-carbohydrate diet, including traditional grain-based vegetarian diets.

How can you tell if you are genetically predisposed to make excess insulin? Take this very simple test: Eat a big pasta meal at lunch and then see how you feel three hours later. If you can barely keep your eyes open, then you are genetically a ticking time bomb. The good news is that the genetic predisposition toward elevated insulin can be controlled by the composition of the food you eat.

Keep in mind that having a genetic predisposition to elevated insulin secretion is very different from having chronically elevated insulin levels, a condition known as *hyperinsulinemia.* If hyperinsuline-mia is diagnosed through a blood test, you have a greatly increased risk of developing diabetes, obesity, cardiovascular disease, and cancer, all of which will decrease your potential longevity. The good news is that the Soy Zone Diet can begin to reverse hyperinsulinemia within a matter of days.

GLUCAGON: THE ANTI-INSULIN HORMONE

In addition to controlling your insulin levels, the Soy Zone Diet can also help you control another hormone called glucagon, which has the opposite effect of insulin. Just like carbohydrates trigger the release of insulin, protein stimulates the release of glucagon.

While insulin is the storage hormone, glucagon is the mobilization hormone: It tells the liver to release stored carbohydrate to maintain blood glucose levels to the brain. Without a constant and consistent supply of blood glucose, the brain will simply shut down and stop func-tioning. If you've ever experienced the light-headedness and shakiness caused by hypoglycemia (low blood sugar levels), then you know how much your brain relies on food to function. When you're hypo-glycemic, your brain virtually commands you to eat any carbohydrate in sight to increase blood sugar levels. Most people describe these as car-bohydrate cravings.

What you may not realize, though, is that the more carbohydrates you eat, the more likely you are to become hypoglycemic. Too many carbohydrates can cause excessive amounts of insulin to be released. As a result, your blood sugar levels dip far below what they were before you had your meal. This leads you on a search for more carbohydrates, which puts you in a vicious cycle.

Eating more protein is the best way to get a handle on hypo-glycemia because protein stimulates the release of glucagon, which maintains blood sugar levels in the brain. What's more, glucagon acts like a hormonal brake that inhibits insulin secretion. So by maintaining relative constant levels of glucagon, you will control insulin levels with far greater ease.

By spreading your protein intake throughout the day, you will constantly produce adequate (but not excessive) amounts of glucagon throughout the day on the Soy Zone. At the same time, you'll never eat too much protein at one meal. Why is this important? First of all, the body can't store excess protein, so whatever it can't use immediately is converted to fat. In addition, excess protein does stimulate the release of insulin, even though this effect is excess slight compared to carbohydrates. The bottom line is that any excess protein you eat over the course of the day, or even at a single meal, will make it harder to reach your hormonal goal, which is optimal insulin control. Eating a balanced amount of protein to carbohydrate at every meal and snack—by following the Soy Zone—will give you a healthy ratio of insulin and glucagon in your bloodstream for the next four to six hours.

THE HORMONAL BENEFITS OF REDUCING CALORIES

The amount of calories you eat also plays a key role in determining your insulin levels. Eating too many calories triggers the release of insulin. For this reason, the Soy Zone is designed to enable you to consume the fewest number of calories possible, while maintaining an excellent mental and physical performance. The calories you eat should contain just enough incoming protein to maintain your strength and your immune system and just enough carbohydrates to stimulate the necessary production of insulin needed to deliver nutrients to your cells. Once again, you'll be eating the right balance of calories—not too many and not too few.

Conserving calories has been a key to the extraordinary longevity of the Okinawans. Consuming an excess of carbohydrates or an excess of calories (or both, in the worst-case scenario) will increase your insulin levels, turning the heroic Dr. Jekyll into the evil Mr. Hyde. It's as simple as that.

Remember that your main carbohydrate sources on the Soy Zone Diet are vegetables, which are very-low-density carbohydrates. You'll supplement your vegetable consumption with fruits, which are intermediate in carbohydrate density. Since you're unlikely to overconsume vegetables and fruit, you'll be able to avoid an overproduction of insulin. On the other hand, you can very easily consume too many high-density carbohydrates, such as starches, cereals, breads, and pasta. That's why they are used in moderation on the Soy Zone Diet.

For example, anyone can eat one cup of pasta, but none of us would consume 12 cups of steamed broccoli. Yet both contain the same amount of carbohydrates. Since many of us overconsume pasta and other high-density carbohydrates, I treat them as condiments on the Soy Zone Diet. The table below shows you just how easy it is to eat too many high-density carbohydrates. Each of these foods contains about 10 grams of carbohydrates—yet they all have very different serving sizes.

Volume Comparison of Different Carbohydrates Providing Approximately 10 grams of Carbohydrate

A. Low-density carbohydrates

Broccoli	3 cups
Peppers	2 cups
Zucchini	2 cups
String beans	1 1/2 cups

B. Intermediate-density carbohydrates

Strawberries	1 cup
Peach	1
Orange	1/2
Apple	1/2

C. High-density carbohydrates

Bread	1/2 slice
Cereal	1/4 cup
Pasta	1/4 cup
Rice	1/5 cup

THE USDA FOOD PYRAMID VERSUS
THE SOY ZONE FOOD PYRAMID

Without a doubt, the excessive consumption of high-density carbohydrates is responsible for Americans' soaring insulin levels because most of us over-consume them. Yet, strangely enough, high-density carbohydrates are staples, not only of traditional grain-based vegetarian diets, but of the eating plan promoted by the U.S. Department of Agriculture (USDA), which sets dietary guidelines for the nation to follow. The government has backed itself into a nutritional corner: More Americans are more obese than ever before, yet the government still continues to recommend cereal, breads, and grains, the very things that trigger excess insulin, which makes us fat and keeps us fat. By now, you should realize that the politically correct carbohydrates you are told to eat might not be your best hormonal choices.

Let's briefly examine the recommendations made in the USDA Food Pyramid, and you'll see why they are virtually guaranteed to increase insulin levels and make Americans fatter. The government recommends eating 6 to 11 servings each day of high-density carbohydrates like pasta, rice, and bagels. Using the serving sizes recommended by the USDA, 11 servings of grains amounts to approximately 220 grams of carbohydrates each day. The government also recommends a minimum of three to five small servings of fruits and vegetables per day. Based on 3 USDA-size servings of vegetables, this would be equivalent to about 15 grams of carbohydrate; 2 servings of fruit would be another 20 grams of carbohydrate. If you add up all the carbohydrates, this gives some 255 grams of carbohydrate. That's more than what is contained in $1^1/_4$ cups of table sugar or six candy bars.

On the other hand, the Soy Zone Diet calls for 10 to 15 daily servings of fruits and vegetables (3 times the amount recommended by the government), which contain about 100 grams of carbohydrates. In addition, you can have maybe 2 servings a day of high-density carbohydrates, generating another 40 grams of carbohydrate. Thus, on the Soy Zone Diet you would be eating a larger amount of the vitamin- and mineral-rich fruits and vegetables, but you would eat only about 140 grams of total carbohydrates, which is more than 40 percent less than that recommended by the USDA (see table on page 218).

Comparison of Total Carbohydrate Consumption Following the USDA Food Pyramid or the Soy Zone Diet

	Servings	Grams of Carbohydrate
A. USDA Recommendations		
Grains	11	220
Fruits	2	20
Vegetables	3	15
Total	16	255
B. Soy Zone Recommendations		
Grains	2	40
Fruits	5	50
Vegetables	10	50
Total	17	140

Reducing your carbohydrate consumption by more than 40 percent on the Soy Zone Diet will also give you a similar reduction in insulin secretion. Now take a look at the comparison of the USDA Food Pyramid and Soy Zone Food Pyramid on page 219. You'll quickly see the differences in terms of which foods are emphasized (the ones at the base of each pyramid). You'll also realize why the USDA Food Pyramid is virtually guaranteed to increase insulin levels; as a result, you'll get fatter, be more likely to develop heart disease, and have a higher risk of premature death.

If the Okinanwan diet was illustrated in a food pyramid format, it would be virtually identical to the Soy Food Pyramid. Considering that your goal is to lead a longer and better life through better insulin control, it should be obvious which of the two food pyramids leads you there.

Comparison of Food Pyramids

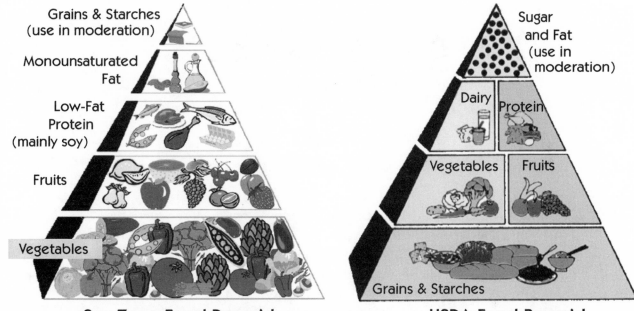

Soy Zone Food Pyramid

Grains & Starches (use in moderation)

Monounsaturated Fat

Low-Fat Protein (mainly soy)

Fruits

Vegetables

USDA Food Pyramid

Sugar and Fat (use in moderation)

Dairy

Protein

Vegetables

Fruits

Grains & Starches

10

Soy Science

Without a doubt, soy has become a hot food trend. Most Americans know about soy and are intrigued by it. Newspaper headlines have played up the benefits of soy to the point that soy products are now viewed as having almost mystical powers to prevent the most common and feared diseases. Study after study have indicated that certain populations throughout the world who consume large amounts of soy protein have a decreased incidence of chronic diseases. As I mentioned in Chapter 1, the health benefits of soy protein include:

- decreased cholesterol levels

- decreased risk of heart disease

- decreased risk of cancer (breast and prostate)

- decreased likelihood of osteoporosis

- decreased symptoms of menopause

The truth is, soy is no magic potion. I'm not trying to sell you an elixir that "works even though we don't know how." Researchers have a fairly clear idea why soy works to prevent disease. Actual molecular mechanisms lie behind soy's magic and have a dramatic impact on the way your body functions. That's why I feel this chapter is so important. Many people shy away from science, but I feel that it's crucial to know a little bit about the soy foods you're putting into your body. After all, soy works like a powerful drug, and it's nice to know something about the drug you're taking. If you don't take the time to learn the fundamentals, you'll be taking a blind leap of faith.

SOY PROTEIN: ITS INSULIN-LOWERING EFFECTS

The unique effects of soy protein on both insulin and glucagon make the Soy Zone the most powerful version of my Zone technology. Like all proteins, soy protein is composed of building blocks called *amino acids*. Some of these amino acids are essential (which means you need to get them from your diet) and others are nonessential (which means your body can manufacture them on its own). Essential amino acids trigger the release of insulin from the pancreas, and soy has a much lower amount of essential amino acids than animal protein. This means that soy protein doesn't raise insulin levels as much as animal protein does. (Compared to carbohydrates, both soy and animal protein have a small effect on insulin levels. It's just that soy has an even smaller effect than animal protein.)

Having such a slight effect on insulin levels means that soy protein can also cause a reduction in cholesterol levels. This is because insulin activates the key enzyme that stimulates cholesterol production in your body. Thus, a decrease in insulin secretion will result in a decrease in the activity of this enzyme and a corresponding decrease in cholesterol.

Like other forms of protein, soy protein stimulates the release of glucagon, the anti-insulin hormone that I discussed in the last chapter. The unique amino acid composition of soy protein stimulates the release of glucagon to a higher degree than animal protein. Glucagon mobilizes stored carbohydrates from the liver to keep the brain supplied with a constant supply of energy, thereby eliminating fatigue and hunger. In addition, increased levels of glucagon inhibit the secretion of insulin because these two hormones constantly regulate each other. Soy's one-two punch of a decreased secretion of insulin and an increased secretion of glucagon results in more controlled insulin levels. That's why soy works better than other forms of protein at balancing your insulin and getting you into the Zone.

Based primarily on the cholesterol-lowering ability of soy protein, the U.S. government has recently recommended the consumption of at least 25 grams per day of soy protein to reduce both total cholesterol and LDL cholesterol, which can lower the risk of heart disease. While I applaud this step, I don't think it goes far enough. Most of the clinical studies that the government's recommendation are based upon involved the consumption of 30 to 60 grams per day of soy protein. Following the Soy Zone Diet, you consume nearly twice as much soy protein as recommended by the government—an amount consistent with the actual clinical research.

A Brief History of the Soybean

Soybeans most likely originated in China some two thousand years ago. The versatility of the soybean is due to its unique composition (42 percent protein, 33 percent carbohydrate, and 20 percent fat) and its extraordinarily high protein content as a plant source. These qualities led to the development of soy milk and tofu and eventually to various fermented forms of soybeans, such as tempeh, which still remain the protein staples of the Asian diet.

Benjamin Franklin apparently introduced soybeans to America when he sent seedlings from Le Jardin des Plantes in Paris to eight farmers in Pennsylvania. Not much happened to these seedlings, since the climate of Pennsylvania is not very suitable for growing soybeans. Fortunately, more soybeans arrived in America as the China trade increased—not as cargo, but as ballast for ships arriving from China. From these humble beginnings, soybeans have emerged as the number-two cash crop in America, a $13 billion-a-year agribusiness with some 62 million acres devoted to growing soybeans. Although nearly 50 percent of all soybeans in the world are produced in America, more than one-third of the soybean crop is sent overseas (primarily to Japan).

The interest in soybeans as a meat substitute in America originated with the Seventh Day Adventists (who stress a vegetarian lifestyle), but the concept didn't take off at first because the first prototypes tasted terrible. With the development of new edible oil-processing technology in the 1920s, soybeans became a valuable commodity as a source of vegetable oil. Today, soybean oil is the number one edible oil used in the United States.

Although oil production was the economic force that drove soybean production in the past, the by-products of soybean oil processing (such as soy protein) have also become increasingly valuable. Initially, soy protein provided an inexpensive source of high-quality protein for animal feed. More recently, soy protein has become a major food ingredient because of its health benefits, which are supported by epidemiological studies.

ADVANCED SOY SCIENCE: ISOFLAVONES

There is no question that eating more soy protein is associated with greater health and longevity. All the benefits of soy protein, however, cannot be fully attributed to its unique amino acid composition. Soy protein is also rich in phytochemicals known as isoflavones, and these substances may have unique disease-fighting powers. Like many micronutrients hailed as magic bullets, isoflavones have been isolated and put into pill form. Before you start popping isoflavone pills, fortified candy bars, or chewing gum, however, you should know a little bit about how isoflavones work and how they amplify the benefits of soy protein.

The two primary isoflavones in soy protein are genistein and daidzein. These two phytochemicals mimic the effects of estrogen in your body. Since they can actually bind to estrogen receptors found on cells, these two isoflavones are known as phytoestrogens. In fact, researchers have found that women who eat a significant amount of soybeans, soy milk, tofu, and tempeh (which are all rich in phytoestrogens) have an easier transition through menopause because they have fewer side effects like hot flashes and mood swings. They concluded that eating 20 grams of soy protein per day provides a modest decrease in the severity of menopausal symptoms. The study's leaders theorize that phytoestrogens mimic the effect of natural estrogens, and this widely publicized finding has generated much of the recent interest in soy. (These results, however, have yet to be confirmed by follow-up studies.)

Although phytoestrogens are about 200 times weaker than natural estrogens, they can have an impact if you consume enough of them. For instance, Japanese women, who eat a great deal of soy, have blood concentrations of these phytoestrogens nearly 1,000 times higher than American females. Not by accident, Japanese women have a much lower rate of hot flashes and other symptoms during menopause.

These same phytoestrogens may have a potential role in reducing osteoporosis. Daidzein is similar in chemical structure to one of the newest drugs (ipriflavone) used to prevent bone loss after menopause. In fact, a 1996 study of women who consumed 40 grams of soy protein isolate containing isoflavones per day found that these women experienced an increase in their bone mass.

The beneficial effects of isoflavones go far beyond their role as phytoestrogens. Isoflavones also act as endocrine disrupters, which means they disrupt other hormonal signals that can turn normal cells into cancerous ones. For example, prostate cancer tumors grow in the presence of the hormone dihydrotestosterone, which is formed from testosterone. Genistein indirectly inhibits the production of dihydrotestosterone, stopping prostate cancer in its tracks. This may explain why Japanese men have a much lower mortality rate from prostate cancer than American men.

Genistein also inhibits the detrimental effects that excess insulin can have on the growth of cancer cells. It appears that genistein stops the signals that insulin (and other tumor-promoting growth hormones) sends out to target cells. When genistein disrupts these messages, target cells never get the message that they should turn cancerous. Because of the ability of genistein to inhibit these signaling pathways, it can decrease your likelihood of cancer.

Thus, soy has three major benefits:

- Through its unique amino acid composition, soy protein can keep insulin levels from becoming elevated, which can reduce the risk of heart disease, diabetes, and certain cancers.

- Soy's rich content of isoflavones, which act like phytoestrogens, can reduce menopausal symptoms like hot flashes and may help reduce the likelihood of osteoporosis.

- These same isoflavones can squelch the hormonal impact of any excess insulin by disrupting the signaling pathways used by insulin and other tumor-promoting hormones. This action reduces the risk of prostate cancer and other cancers. The hormone disruption also explains why soy doesn't increase breast cancer risk even though it acts like an estrogen—which can stimulate breast cancer cells. Genistein inhibits the action of breast cancer tumors by disrupting their signaling pathways, which outweighs the negative effect of the breast cell stimulation.

Yet with all of these potential benefits, I don't recommend taking isoflavone supplements because I think that—like any food or drug—too much is never a good thing. In high amounts, isoflavones may have potential negative effects on other hormones, especially in terms of thyroid function. Some preliminary studies suggest that excess isoflavones can adversely affect the binding of thyroid hormones, which can lead to an underactive thyroid function. (Isoflavones can also bind to the thyroid receptor just as they can bind to the estrogen receptor. This inhibits the binding of your thyroid hormones so you may induce a hypothyroid condition, which can cause weight gain and lethargy.)

Another concern about excess isoflavone consumption involves the potential acceleration of brain aging in elderly males. Recent research from the ongoing Honolulu Heart Study suggests a link between tofu consumption and the loss of cognitive ability and decreased brain weight in elderly males. It may be that the overconsumption of phyto-estrogens has a potentially adverse effect on male brains. This would not be the first time that an adverse effect has been observed in males who are getting too much estrogen. For example, when men took estro-gen pills to see if they could reduce their heart attack risk in studies done in the early 1970s, they actually experienced an increased risk of heart attack.

I'm not concerned that you will get too many isoflavones on the Soy Zone, but I do feel that these preliminary research results should deter you from taking isoflavone supplements. What's more, soy protein con-taining isoflavones is known to reduce cholesterol levels, yet this effect isn't seen in people who consume isolated isoflavone supplements. It appears that isoflavones need to be consumed with soy protein in order to exert their cardiovascular and hormonal benefits. There could also be an unknown factor in soy that works with isoflavones to bring about health benefits.

As more and more products containing large amounts of isolated isoflavones appear on the shelves of pharmacies and health food stores, well-respected researchers have become alarmed. For example, Herman Adlecreutz, a pioneer in isoflavone research, has stated, "I am myself frightened a little bit by all of this. There is so much we don't know."

I agree with his sentiments, which is why I am against isoflavone supplementation in pill form until more research is completed about the benefits and risks of large amounts of isoflavones. I do, however, feel comfortable recommending that you eat large amounts of soy protein.

If you're concerned about overconsuming isoflavones, a good com-promise is this: Eat one-third of your soy protein from soy products that contain no phytoestrogens. These products include virtually all of the soybean meat substitutes, and contain no phytoestrogens because they are made from alcohol-extracted soy protein concentrates. Traditional soy protein products (tofu, soy beans, soy milk, tempeh, soy nuts, soy flour, soy grits, and textured soy protein) have the highest con-centration of isoflavones, and soy protein isolate powders have about half the amount of isoflavones found in traditional soy products.

How the Soy Zone Diet Stacks Up Against the Traditional Vegetarian Diet

Many people become vegetarians because they want to live a longer and healthier life. The primary health benefits of a traditional grain-based vegetarian diet are usually attributed to a reduction in fat, cholesterol, and protein along with an increased intake of fiber, antioxidants, and phytochemicals. The question is: Are these perceived health benefits supported by the research? Not really. Although vegetarians do derive health benefits from an increased consumption of vegetables and fruit, they are making grave health mistakes by not consuming enough protein and monounsaturated fat. What's more, they consume way too many carbohydrates in the form of high-density grains. All these carbohydrates add up to one thing: elevated insulin levels. (And you know all the problems this can cause.)

Let's examine each of the stated health claims for traditional grain-based vegetarian diets to see how they stack up against the Soy Zone Diet.

HEALTH CLAIM #1: VEGETARIANS EAT LESS FAT

You may have heard again and again that dietary fat is the underlying cause of all disease. The truth is, there are very little data to support that belief. In fact, in a review article published in 1998 in *The New England*

227

Journal of Medicine, three of the top nutritional researchers in the world analyzed the major long-term studies on low-fat, high-carbohydrate diets. Their conclusions can be summarized by the following quotes:

> Replacement of fat by carbohydrates has not been shown to reduce the risk of heart disease.
>
> Beneficial effects of high-carbohydrate diets on the risk of cancer or on body weight also have not been substantiated.

So after reviewing all the published literature, these researchers found no apparent relationship between dietary fat intake and chronic diseases such as obesity, heart disease, and cancer.

It turns out that dietary fat alone doesn't make you fat. It is excess insulin that makes you fat and keeps you fat (remember the Jekyll-and-Hyde effect from Chapter 9). Vegetarians (as well as non-vegetarians) who consume grain-based diets composed primarily of high-density carbohydrates, such as starches, grains, and pasta, have the potential to become overweight without eating significant amounts of fat. This is because they produce too much insulin. This very same excess insulin also puts them at higher risk of developing heart disease, Type 2 diabetes, and cancer.

Unlike traditional grain-based vegetarian diets, the primary sources of carbohydrates on the Soy Zone Diet are vegetables and fruits. Switching to these lower-density carbohydrate sources reduces insulin levels, because it is very difficult to overconsume them. In addition, the Soy Zone Diet supplies higher amounts of soy protein, which stimulates the hormone glucagon. Glucagon acts as a powerful inhibitor of insulin secretion, while simultaneously maintaining blood sugar levels so that you aren't hungry or mentally fatigued between meals.

It's important to realize that it's not fat *per se* that causes heart disease, but often the consumption of the wrong type of fat. Although the absolute level of dietary fat in the Soy Zone Diet is similar to a traditional grain-based vegetarian diet, the composition of the fat is very different. Traditional grain-based diets get most of their fat from grains and seed oils that are often rich in unhealthy Omega-6 fatty acids. The overconsumption of Omega-6 fatty acids can lead to the excess production of arachidonic acid (especially when insulin levels are elevated). Arachidonic acid, in turn, is the building block for "bad" eicosanoids, substances in the body that make platelets aggregate and clot and also depress the immune system. As a result, this sticky blood can cause blockages in the arteries, which can lead to the development of a heart attack or a cancerous tumor. These scientific explanations are explained in greater detail in my previous books *The Zone* and *The Anti-Aging Zone*.

Unlike grain-based vegetarian diets, the Soy Zone Diet emphasizes monounsaturated fat, such as olive oil, as its major fat component, so you get very little Omega-6 fatty acid. What's more, you'll get adequate levels of beneficial Omega-3 fatty acids on the Soy Zone because of supplementation with fish oil or algae oil capsules. As you can see, although vegetarian diets and the Soy Zone Diet contain about the same amount of fat, the Soy Zone has a much healthier balance of Omega-3 to Omega-6 fatty acids.

HEALTH CLAIM #2: VEGETARIANS EAT LESS CHOLESTEROL

Besides declaring a war on fat, Americans have also waged a battle against cholesterol. Not all cholesterol, though, is negatively associated with heart disease. For example, the higher your levels of "good" HDL cholesterol, the lower your risk of having a heart attack. Likewise, the higher your levels of "bad" LDL cholesterol, the more likely it is you will have a heart attack. Based on this information, Americans are spending billions of dollars buying drugs that inhibit "bad" cholesterol formation.

While vegetarians do tend to have lower LDL cholesterol levels, they also have lower HDL cholesterol levels, so they get a mixed bag in terms of their heart disease risk. Moreover, recent studies have shown that elevated insulin levels are far more predictive of heart disease than LDL cholesterol. In fact, triglyceride levels are more predictive than is LDL cholesterol, and elevated triglyceride levels often result from elevated insulin. You can still get the benefit of lowering LDL cholesterol levels following the Soy Zone Diet, but you will receive a far greater impact from reducing excess insulin and triglycerides.

HEALTH CLAIM #3: VEGETARIANS EAT MORE FIBER

Research suggests that eating a diet high in fiber leads to a lower risk of colon cancer. A new finding, however, suggests that fiber alone won't lower your risk. Harvard Medical School researchers found no relation between fiber intake and the appearance of colon cancer in women. Most likely, the negative effect of excess insulin canceled out the benefits of increased fiber consumption. The Soy Zone Diet, with its emphasis on vegetables and fruits, is exceptionally rich in fiber. In fact, you get more fiber than you would on a typical grain-based vegetarian diet, and you won't experience potentially soaring insulin levels. Thus, you actually can reap more of the benefits from fiber following the Soy Zone Diet than on a vegetarian diet.

HEALTH CLAIM #4: VEGETARIANS CONSUME MORE ANTIOXIDANTS

The most studied antioxidant is Vitamin E, and study after study have confirmed its significant health benefits, such as the reduction of free radical formation (which reduces the risk of cancer and heart disease). Unfortunately, all diets contain inadequate levels of Vitamin E, which is found primarily in vegetable oils. Therefore, to get the health benefits of Vitamin E, vegetarians (as well as virtually everyone else) should consume extra Vitamin E supplements.

As far as the other antioxidants go, vegetables and fruits are the best source of these. Grain products, on the other hand, contain very little—if any—antioxidants. Since you eat more vegetables and fruits on the Soy Zone Diet compared to a traditional grain-based diet, you not only get a greater amount of antioxidants, but also a far greater variety.

HEALTH CLAIM #5: VEGETARIANS DON'T OVERCONSUME PROTEIN

No one should ever overconsume protein, because the body will convert any excess protein into fat. However, most vegetarians following a grain-based diet get *too little* protein. This underconsumption of protein can decrease the efficiency of your immune system and may also increase your risk of heart disease. That is the conclusion of a 1999 study from Harvard Medical School that found that women who increased their protein consumption and decreased their carbohydrates (while keeping their total calories and fat intake constant) experienced a 26 percent lower risk of a heart attack.

Unlike vegetarian diets that reduce protein intake dramatically, the Soy Zone Diet is based on your personal protein prescription and spreads that amount of protein throughout the day like the intravenous drip of a drug. Furthermore, the Soy Zone Diet places a great emphasis on soy protein (at least 35–50 grams per day) because of its insulin-lowering effects, plus the additional benefits of isoflavones that can inhibit the adverse effects of elevated insulin. Recall that the Okinawans, who are the longest-lived people in the world, eat approximately 100 grams of soy protein per day.

HEALTH CLAIM #6: VEGETARIANS LIVE LONGER

Vegetarians do live longer than the general population, but how much of their longevity is due to their diet and how much is due to leading a healthier lifestyle in general? Vegetarians tend to be more health-conscious: They exercise more, smoke and drink less, and pay closer attention to their food choices than the general population. These are built-in factors that make it difficult to issue any definitive statements that a vegetarian diet, in and of itself, improves longevity. I don't think anyone would argue that smoking less, drinking less, and exercising more improves health and thus longevity. The real question is: What are the *additional* benefits for health-conscious individuals who follow vegetarian diets? If you include these other lifestyle factors, does following a vegetarian diet still improve longevity compared to the general population?

For the first time, it may be possible to answer that question definitively. In a recent study published in the *British Medical Journal*, researchers followed about 11,000 health-conscious people for more than 17 years, of which about 40 percent were vegetarians. As you might expect, the overall mortality rate of the total group was about 56 percent less than the general population, which is in line with other published studies that included only vegetarians. Once the survival data were adjusted to take into account smoking habits, age, and sex, however, a different picture emerged. Now vegetarians showed *no differences* in overall mortality compared to the general population. Although vegetarians had a 10 percent lower mortality rate from heart disease, this was offset by a 65 percent *increase* in mortality from breast cancer in vegetarian women. Researchers can't explain the increase in breast cancer death rates, but other research has found that the more bread, pasta, and rice you consume, the greater your risk of dying from breast cancer or other cancers.

The only proven way to dramatically increase longevity is by lowering your intake of calories. The Soy Zone Diet is based on the principle of restricting your calories to the point at which you get an optimal intake of protein, fat, and carbohydrates without overconsuming them. Sixty years of compelling research have found that restricting calories increases longevity. Thus the Soy Zone Diet, coupled with a healthy lifestyle, *guarantees* to increase your longevity. Perhaps, not surprisingly, the Okinawan diet discussed in Chapter 2 is very similar to the Soy Zone Diet. And Okinawa produces the largest percentage of individuals reaching age 100 and beyond than any other society in the world.

WHY THE SOY ZONE IS YOUR GREATEST DEFENSE AGAINST HEART DISEASE

The Soy Zone Diet is your best defense against having a heart attack, which means that it's your greatest ally toward living a longer life. It wins hands-down against a grain-based vegetarian diet in terms of reducing your risk of heart disease. These are pretty bold statements, so let's look at the scientific data that support them.

The best way to determine whether a diet can prevent fatal heart attacks is to conduct an intervention study, in which researchers select from a group of people who already have an existing disease (in this case heart disease), and then determine whether or not a dietary intervention prevents patients from dying from that disease. To date, two long-term intervention studies on heart disease patients have been conducted using diet. One was called the Lifestyle Trial, in which patients were put on a very-low-fat, grain-based vegetarian diet coupled with increased exercise and meditation to reduce stress for a five-year period. This study also had a control group who were simply told to follow a low-fat diet that included lean cuts of meat, chicken, and fish and plenty of grains, fruits, and vegetables—an eating plan endorsed by the American Heart Association for heart disease patients.

In the second intervention study, a four-year study known as the Lyon Diet Heart Study, patients who had already suffered a heart attack were placed in two dietary groups. One group ate more fruits and vegetables, had most of their protein coming from legumes (including soy) and fish, used primarily olive oil, and supplemented their diet with additional Omega-3 fatty acids so that nearly 30 percent of the calories were as fat. (Known as the Mediterranean diet, this diet is similar to the Soy Zone Diet in its content of fat and higher amounts of vegetables and fruits. The Mediterranean diet, however, has a lower ratio of protein to carbohydrate than the Soy Zone Diet, so it won't lower insulin as well.) The second group in the Lyon study followed a diet advocated by the American Heart Association. Since the control groups in each of these intervention studies were very similar, we can compare the results to see whether the grain-based vegetarian diet or the Mediterranean diet demonstrated the greatest reduction in the number of fatal heart attacks.

First, let's look at the Lifestyle Trial. The results after five years can be seen in the following table.

Lifestyle Trial Effect on Fatal Heart Attacks	
Group	**Fatal Heart Attacks**
Intervention (n=28 patients)	2
Control (n=20 patients)	1

Given the fact that the patients following the vegetarian diet had twice the number of fatal heart attacks as those in the control group, this is not exactly a ringing endorsement of the high-carbohydrate vegetarian diet used in the Lifestyle Trial. With so small a sample being studied, the results could have been due to chance except for this one thing: The patients on the vegetarian plan experienced a 25 percent increase in their triglyceride-to-HDL cholesterol ratio. This means that their harmful triglyceride levels increased while their protective HDL levels decreased—not a good thing if you're trying to prevent a heart attack. I firmly believe the study's poor results are directly related to this worsening of these lipid levels, a sign that insulin levels have risen as well.

A statement made by well-known cardiologist K. Lance Gould, in a 1996 letter published in the *Journal of the American Medical Association*, backs up my belief:

> Frequently triglyceride levels increase and HDL cholesterol levels decrease for individuals on a vegetarian, high-carbohydrate diet. Since low HDL cholesterol, particularly with high triglycerides incurs substantial risk of coronary events, I do not recommend a high-carbohydrate strict vegetarian diet.

Why this quote is so important is that Gould was one of the lead researchers involved in the highly touted Lifestyle Trial. Obviously, his words are not a resounding support of a high-carbohydrate, low-fat vegetarian diet for cardiovascular patients.

I don't want you to think, however, that dietary interventions are useless for preventing fatal heart attacks. Dietary changes can be extremely helpful, according to the results of the Lyon Diet Heart Study, which were published in 1999 (see table below).

Lyon Diet Trial Effect on Fatal Hearts Attacks	
Group	Fatal Heart Attacks
Intervention (n=303 patients)	6
Control (n=302 patients)	19

As the table on page 234 indicates, people in the intervention group were two-thirds less likely to have a fatal heart attack as their control group counterparts. What's intriguing is that both the intervention and control group ate about the same amount of fat, protein, carbohydrates, and calories. The major difference between the two groups rested on the type of fat they consumed. The control group had an increased intake of Omega-6 fatty acids (the heart-damaging kind found in vegetable oils), whereas the intervention group ate a lot of fish rich in long-chain Omega-3 fatty acids (the heart-healthy kind), in addition to supplements with extra short-chain Omega-3 fatty acids.

What's clear, though, is how much more effective the Lyon intervention diet was at preventing fatal heart attacks than the Lifestyle intervention diet. The levels of fat consumption and type of fat in the Lyon diet closely resembled the levels found in the Okinawan diet (approximately 30 percent of calories as fat). What's more, the Lyon diet had a much higher protein-to-carbohydrate ratio than the vegetarian Lifestyle diet, which is carbohydrate-rich. The higher protein-to-carbohydrate ratio in the Lyon study probably led to a reduction in insulin levels, which has been found to provide protection against heart disease.

Yet, as impressive as the Lyon Diet Heart Study was, I believe the benefits would have been even greater if the patients had followed the Soy Zone Diet. Why? Because the Soy Zone Diet would have provided an even better protein-to-carbohydrate ratio than the Lyon Diet Heart Study, and would have lowered insulin even more. In addition, a greater proportion of the protein would have come primarily from soy protein, which has less of a stimulating effect on insulin than animal protein does. The Soy Zone Diet would also have been richer in long-chain Omega-3 fatty acids because of supplementation with fish oils or algae oils. Finally, the Soy Zone Diet includes more fruits and vegetables, which are also known to lower the risk of heart disease. Just consider this: If the Soy Zone Diet yields even better results than the Lyon Diet Heart Study, you will gain even more protection against heart disease, just like the Okinawans.

Let me state emphatically that this chapter was not intended to bash vegetarian diets. I don't really think in terms of "good" or "bad" diets. It's only a question of which diet will do the best job of control-ling your own insulin levels most effectively. You can get this answer by having your blood insulin levels tested. As I mentioned earlier in the book, your blood doesn't lie and it doesn't have a political agenda. The results of your longevity report card, described in Chapter 8, will let you know how you are doing whatever your diet might be.

Frequently Asked Questions

12

GENERAL

Does being on the Soy Zone Diet mean that I must avoid all animal protein?

Absolutely not. Unless you're a vegetarian and wish to abstain from all forms of animal protein, you can certainly include fish, chicken, meat, and low-fat dairy products in the Soy Zone Diet. Try to consume at least half your daily protein intake in the form of soy protein. This means about 40 grams of soy protein per day for the average female and 50 grams of soy protein per day for the average male. You can mix and match Zone meals with Soy Zone meals. For instance, if you're a vegetarian who eats eggs and dairy products, you can top a soy veggie burger with low-fat cheese or make tofu scrambled eggs (with egg whites). If you're not a vegetarian, you can incorporate poultry, fish, and lean cuts of beef into your Zone meals. In fact, I recommend having one fish meal a day (preferably tuna, salmon, or another dark-fleshed fish) to get a healthy dose of long-chain Omega-3 fatty acids.

Why is the balance of protein to carbohydrate so important for every Soy Zone meal and snack?

Hormonally, you're only as good as your last meal, and hormonally you're only as good as your next meal. Therefore, the balance of protein to carbohydrate at each meal will determine both your insulin and glucagon levels for the next four to six hours. Eat too many carbohydrates and not enough protein at a meal, and insulin levels will increase too much. Eat too few carbohydrates and too much protein at a meal, and your insulin levels will be too depressed. What you are searching for is a continuous balance, and that can only be achieved by maintaining a relatively constant protein-to-carbohydrate ratio from meal to meal.

Why is excess insulin so harmful?

Excess insulin is the primary accelerator of the aging process. It is also the primary risk factor associated with increased cardiovascular disease. Many of the physical signs of aging, such as sagging skin, obesity, decreased strength, decreased mental focus, and increased risk of chronic disease, are directly or indirectly related to increased insulin levels. Of course, without enough insulin, your cells would starve to death, because insulin drives nutrients into cells. Therefore, you need to maintain a zone of insulin: not too high, not too low. The only drug known to medical science that can maintain insulin in an appropriate zone— enough to deliver nutrients to cells, yet not accelerate aging—is food.

Which comes first, excess insulin or obesity?

Until recently there were no good data to answer that question. Now recent long-term studies have demonstrated that excess insulin levels precede the development of obesity. Likewise, it is well known that insulin levels drop dramatically before any change in weight is observed.

The Soy Zone Diet only contains about 1,200 calories a day for women and 1,500 calories a day for men. Isn't this too little to live on?

Actually, you'll maximize your chances of living longer on the Soy Zone plan precisely because you're restricting your calorie intake. Eating fewer calories lowers your insulin levels and prevents the formation of free radicals (which can destroy healthy cells and accelerate aging). I realize that many weight-loss plans put people on 1,200- to 1,500-calorie-per-day diets that leave them feeling famished all the time. The Soy Zone is different because you're consuming adequate amounts of protein and fat without overconsuming carbohydrates. As a result, you don't feel hungry between meals because you are maintaining your blood sugar levels. So on fewer calories, you'll consume adequate levels of protein to maintain your muscle mass and immune system and adequate levels of vitamins and minerals (primarily found in vegetables and fruits). Make sure you get adequate amounts of long-chain Omega-3 fatty acids, either through fish consumption or supplements of fish or algae oil, and you've got all the nutrition your body needs.

Why is the Zone Diet so controversial?

Beats me. The Zone Diet is based on two words: balance and moderation. You balance the ratio of protein to carbohydrate, and eat moderate amounts of calories at every meal. So it certainly can't be that aspect of the Zone Diet that is controversial. Furthermore, the Zone Diet is based on what your grandmother told you to eat two generations ago: (1) Eat small meals throughout the day; (2) have some protein at every meal; (3) always eat your fruits and vegetables; and (4) take your cod-liver oil (a good source of long-chain Omega-3 fatty acids). Obviously, that aspect of the Zone Diet can't be controversial.

In my opinion, the reason the Zone Diet is controversial is that it forces people to think of the hormonal consequences of food instead of thinking only about calories and fat. What's more, the media has, on several occasions, lumped the Zone Diet together with high-protein diets that advocate eating all the steak, fried eggs, and bacon that you want (while avoiding fruits and vegetables). Anyone familiar with the Zone Diet knows that it is not a high-protein diet, nor does it allow you to eat endless amounts of any food. I think this misinterpretation of the Zone Diet has led to much of the unwarranted criticism.

Should I avoid products made from genetically modified soybeans?

Nothing is more controversial than this topic. Plants, including soybeans, have been genetically modified for hundreds of years by crossbreeding. Cloning technology has simply accelerated the process by allowing the insertion of genetic material that makes the soybeans more resistant to pesticides. More than one-third of all soybeans grown in the U.S. last year were genetically modified. Critics of genetically modified organisms (GMOs) say that these products were rushed to market without adequately testing them for human safety. They worry that there are hidden health risks to humans.

I personally have not seen any data that would suggest that genetically modified soybeans pose any danger to humans, especially in soy meat substitutes or isolated protein powders, because of the extensive processing that is done to the soybean to make those products. However, if you have a concern, you can purchase soy foods that have a non-GMO label on them. Be prepared, though, to find a more limited availability, especially among the more modern soy products, such as soy meat substitutes.

Wasn't man designed to be a vegetarian?

On the contrary, man has always eaten meat. In the beginning of human history, man's primary source of protein came from scavenging dead animals. With the appearance of modern man (*homo sapiens*) some 100,000 years ago, intelligence levels increased as we began to eat shellfish rich in the long-chain Omega-3 fatty acid DHA. Once man became a proficient hunter, he consumed some 200 to 300 grams of animal protein per day. Faced with potential starvation caused by his overhunting of big game species, mankind turned to the development of agriculture some 10,000 years ago. Starches and grains provided the most calories with the least amount of physical labor to feed a growing population. But these foods, unfortunately, provided a much lower protein and higher carbohydrate intake than he had consumed during the previous 90,000 years of eating low-fat animal protein, vegetables, and fruits. Anthropologists have found that the skeletal remains of hunter-gatherers show fewer signs of disease than the remains of the early farmers.

How destructive is agriculture to the environment?

All agriculture is ultimately destructive to the environment; only hunter-gatherer societies are truly enviro-friendly. However, because of the great amounts of grain required to produce animal feed, the beef and chicken industries now have a far more negative impact on the landscape than does soybean production. For this reason, using soybean meat substitutes and protein powders can dramatically decrease the ecological impact of providing enough protein to maintain optimal health for the world's rapidly growing population.

What is the difference between a vegan and a lacto-ovo vegetarian?

Vegans will not eat any dairy or egg products, whereas a lacto-ovo vegetarian will eat both dairy and egg products. Since both low-fat egg and dairy products provide excellent sources of protein, a lacto-ovo vegetarian diet provides a far greater variety of protein sources than a vegan's diet. In the past, the number of protein-rich sources for a vegan was limited to primarily tofu. But with the advent of new technology (especially soy meat substitutes), a far greater number of food products are available that give the vegan virtually as many protein possibilities as a lacto-ovo vegetarian has.

Are there any particular vitamins and minerals that vegetarians need to get through supplements?

Long-chain Omega-3 fatty acids are probably the most important supplement, because you can't get adequate amounts of these vital fatty acids unless you eat significant amounts of fish. The other vitamin that everyone needs in greater amounts, regardless of his or her diet, is Vitamin E. It is simply impossible to get enough Vitamin E to obtain the proven health benefits without supplementation. In addition, vegetarians (especially vegans) should consider supplementing their diets with vitamin B12, which is found primarily in animal protein sources. Vitamin B12 is important for preventing the overproduction of homocysteine, a chemical that can damage arteries and for the proper functioning of nerve cells. You should also consider taking a multivitamin if you're not eating enough servings of fruits and vegetables (like the ten to fifteen servings per day recommended on the Soy Zone Diet).

What is the nutritional difference between raw food versus cooked food?

Proponents of raw food believe that the enzymes contained in raw food are required for adequate digestion and that cooking destroys these enzymes, which makes the food less digestible. In reality, the opposite is true. Cooking breaks down the structure of cell walls, making them more digestible by the body's own digestive enzymes. Obviously, you can overcook food and destroy many of the vitamins and lose many of the minerals. Therefore, the best compromise is to lightly steam vegetables. Most fruits are usually eaten raw anyway. All grains (which are minimal components of the Soy Zone Diet) must be thoroughly cooked or processed in order to be digested.

PROTEIN

Why does the body need protein?

You are constantly losing protein, and it needs to be replenished by the diet to maintain your body's equilibrium. Your immune system, your muscles, and the enzymes that make your body run smoothly are all composed of protein. If you're not consuming adequate dietary protein, your body will start tearing down muscle to provide the necessary amino acids to keep the system going. This is like tearing down the front of your house in order to build the back—not a very smart idea.

What are essential amino acids?

There are twenty amino acids used to make protein. Nine of them can't be made by the human body and therefore must be supplied by the diet. If there is an inadequate level of any one of these nine essential amino acids, the body's ability to make new protein required for enzymes and your immune system will be compromised.

If I'm a vegetarian, is there a need to combine vegetable proteins at each meal?

Many vegetable sources of protein are deficient in at least one of the nine essential amino acids. Therefore, it was originally thought that each meal had to combine various sources to get a complete spectrum of amino acids. For example, you might have to eat beans with rice. It turns out that the body has a circulating pool of amino acids, so that as long as you get adequate levels of each essential amino acid in the course of the day, you won't have any problems. This gives vegetarians far greater latitude when constructing meals. In addition, soy meat substitutes and, in particular, soy protein isolates provide a more complete spectrum of essential amino acids, thus making them great vegetarian sources to ensure adequate daily intake of essential amino acids.

Are protein requirements constant during your life?

No. In fact, they are much higher at birth for the newborn and slightly higher for the elderly (based on body weight) than they are for a young adult.

Is there a difference between the way your body absorbs animal protein versus vegetable protein?

Yes, vegetable protein sources have a much higher fiber content, and much of the protein is embedded in this fiber network. As a result, only 70 percent of the actual protein is absorbed from vegetable sources like soybeans, regular beans, and legumes. Processed soy foods (like tofu and soy meat substitutes), on the other hand, contain very little fiber, so virtually all of the protein they contain is absorbed.

Why are soybeans unique?

Soybeans are probably the most versatile food on earth because they contain high amounts of both protein and fat relative to carbohydrates. Unlike typical beans and legumes, soybeans actually contain more protein than carbohydrate, and therefore become an integral component of Soy Zone meals.

Do different protein sources have different effects on insulin?

Here, I believe, is the real benefit of soybeans. Because of its unique amino acid composition, soy protein has a much lesser impact on insulin secretion and a greater one on stimulation of glucagon than animal protein. The ability of soy protein to simultaneously reduce insulin secretion and increase glucagon secretion may account for many of the medical benefits of increased soybean consumption, such as decreased cholesterol synthesis and improved cardiovascular health.

How are modern soy products produced?

The first modern soybean product was defatted soy flour, developed in the 1920s from the residue left after the oil is extracted from the soybean. Defatted soy flour contains about 50 percent protein by weight and is still used extensively in the food industry (and especially the animal food industry). Soy flour led to the development of textured soy protein, also known as textured vegetable protein (TVP). Extracting soy flour with alcohol makes soy protein concentrate, which is higher in soy protein, containing approximately 70 percent protein by weight. This process, however, also removes the beneficial isoflavones, which have numerous health benefits.

The latest generation of soy products is called *soy protein isolates*. These products come from soy flour, from which excess carbohydrates are removed by water, thus preserving many of the beneficial isoflavones. Soy protein isolates have the highest levels of protein (more than 90 percent), and retain approximately 50 percent of the isoflavones found in the original soybean.

What types of food products can be made from soybeans?

Virtually anything, now that various types of soy protein powders are available. The first generation of soybean-derived products was soy milk and tofu, first produced more than 1,000 years ago. With new forms of soy protein powder, it is now possible to make a great variety of meat and dairy substitute products.

How is tofu made?

In many ways, tofu is the vegan equivalent of cottage cheese. Whereas cottage cheese comes from milk, tofu is derived from soy milk. Soy milk is the liquid that is produced from pressing ground soybeans that have been briefly simmered. Magnesium chloride is added to the soy milk, which separates the soy milk into curds and whey. The precipitated curds are formed into blocks, which are termed tofu. A similar process is used to make cottage cheese from milk.

What is the difference between silken tofu and firm tofu?

The whey is not removed from silken tofu during manufacturing and is blended back into the curds. This gives silken tofu a smoother, more custard-like texture than block tofu. This type of tofu is preferred in Japanese cooking. Traditional tofu has the whey removed, and the curds are pressed into blocks. This is the type of tofu used in Chinese cooking. Commercially, tofu is pressed into blocks with various amounts of water. As more water is removed from the curds, more carbohydrate is also removed. Therefore, soft tofu has a lower protein density and slightly more carbohydrate than either firm or extra-firm tofu. Because of the lower levels of carbohydrate relative to protein and higher protein densities, I recommend using firm or extra-firm tofu in the Soy Zone Diet.

What is the difference between tofu and tempeh?

Mixing a certain mold (*rhizopus oligosporas*) with cooked soybeans creates tempeh. The mold produces a fibrous network that holds the soy protein together. Tempeh is usually more protein-rich than cooked soybeans, but still has a higher carbohydrate content than tofu. The texture of tempeh is a little more difficult to work with than tofu, but it is very versatile. Tempeh is used extensively in Indonesian cooking.

After reading the food labels of pasta, rice, and bread, I've noticed that these products contain some protein. Am I getting a substantial amount?

Although many traditional vegetarian foods contain protein, they tend to contain negligible amounts of protein compared to their carbohydrate content. Grains and starches have such large amounts of carbohydrates that any beneficial hormonal effect from their protein content is virtually nil. Even beans and legumes, which are relatively rich in protein, still contain an abundance of carbohydrates compared to protein. Soybeans, however, are the only bean or legume that have a higher amount of absorbable protein relative to carbohydrate. Some vegetables such as broccoli have a good ratio of protein-to-carbohydrate, but they contain such small amounts of protein per serving that it's impractical to use them as your primary source of protein. With the new generation of soy meat substitutes, you can very easily obtain adequate levels of high-quality protein with far lesser volumes of food.

Does animal protein cause cancer?

No. In fact, Harvard Medical School researchers have shown that women with breast cancer have a greater chance for survival if they eat more protein. There is, however, an association between red meat and prostate cancer in males. This is because most red meat in this country is also very fatty, containing high percentages of a certain Omega-6 polyunsaturated fatty acid known as arachidonic acid. Arachidonic acid, known to accelerate cancer, is not present in vegetable protein sources.

There is a stronger link between excess insulin levels and cancer. This is because excess insulin can make the body produce more arachidonic acid even though you are not eating any animal protein. Recent studies have indicated that breast, stomach, and colon cancers are associated with increased starch consumption, which can increase insulin levels. On the other hand, eating lots of fruits and vegetables has always been correlated with a lower cancer risk. One very simple reason may be that it's difficult to overconsume carbohydrates if you are eating fruits and vegetables. If you don't overconsume carbohydrates, then it is difficult to overproduce insulin. And if you don't overproduce insulin, you will make less arachidonic acid.

Does eating animal protein cause osteoporosis?

No, despite that constant refrain from some nutritional camps. In neo-Paleolithic times, the average protein consumption was estimated to be 200 to 300 grams per day, and there is no evidence of any osteoporosis found in skeletal remains from this period. Furthermore, a recent study has demonstrated that postmenopausal women who have the highest intakes of protein have a 70 percent lower risk of having a hip fracture.

Why do high-protein diets fail?

Unlike the Soy Zone Diet, which contains a balance of protein and carbohydrates (with actually more carbohydrates than protein), high-proteins diets are just that—excessive levels of protein and almost no carbohydrates. These high-protein diets generate an abnormal metabolic state known as ketosis, which occurs when there isn't enough carbohydrate in the diet and the body is unable to completely metabolize stored fat. The incomplete metabolism of fat produces chemicals known as ketone bodies, and the body will go to great strides to eliminate them through increased urination. Unfortunately, increased urination also causes the loss of electrolytes such as potassium, which gives rise to both fatigue and irritability. Another short-term consequence of high-protein diets is the tearing down of muscle mass to make adequate levels of glucose for the brain. If insufficient carbohydrate is coming from the diet, the brain will instruct the body's muscles to begin consuming themselves and turn this protein into enough carbohydrate to maintain brain function.

Although millions of people have lost weight on high-protein diets, the same millions have invariably regained all the lost weight. Why? If you stay in ketosis for weeks or months, your fat cells adapt to this state and begin to sequester and hold onto their fat stores. In essence, continued ketosis causes your fat cells to become fat magnets. Moreover, continually eating high levels of saturated fat, found in many animal protein sources, will eventually lead not only to cardiovascular problems, but also a condition called insulin resistance where your cells become less responsive to insulin. With time, insulin levels increase in the bloodstream and rapid weight gain can occur. This is because excess insulin caused the accumulation of body fat in the first place. Finally, new research has demonstrated that continued ketosis causes oxidation of your lipoproteins, which is one of the major factors in the development of heart disease.

CARBOHYDRATES

What are the differences between complex carbohydrates and simple carbohydrates?

Complex carbohydrates are merely simple carbohydrates (primarily glucose) that are held together by relatively weak chemical bonds. These chemical bonds are quickly broken down during digestion, turning any complex carbohydrate into a simple carbohydrate, since the body can only absorb simple carbohydrates. Items such as grains, breads, and starches are examples of complex carbohydrates that are rapidly turned into simple sugars. Complex carbohydrates are broken down mainly into glucose and fructose. The simple carbohydrate glucose enters the bloodstream very quickly, whereas fructose, the simple carbohydrate found in fruit, must slowly be converted into glucose in the liver before it can enter the bloodstream. Therefore, some simple carbohydrate foods like fruit actually enter the bloodstream as glucose (blood sugar) at a much slower rate than many complex carbohydrates composed of glucose chains, such as starches. In fact, table sugar, which is composed of equal parts of glucose and fructose, enters the bloodstream at a slower rate than a puffed rice cake.

Are grains essential to human health?

Not really. In fact, 10,000 years ago there were no grains on the face of the earth. Before the advent of agriculture, the only carbohydrates available to mankind were fruits and vegetables, and hence our genes were adapted for this type of low-density carbohydrate consumption. Many people don't have genes that were adapted to eating higher-density carbohydrates, such as grains and grain-derived products (pasta, bagels, breads, cereals, etc.). However, eating certain grains (especially oatmeal and barley, which are rich in soluble fiber) in small amounts is a great addition to any diet. This is because they are rich in soluble fiber, which slows their entry rate into the bloodstream, thereby lowering the overall insulin response. Moreover, eating excess grains (even oatmeal and barley) is a sure way to increase insulin and minimize the health benefits of any diet.

Does eating more fruits and vegetables prevent heart disease and cancer?

Yes, but I believe not for the reasons usually given. It is often assumed that the vitamins and other phytochemicals (such as beta-carotene) found in fruits and vegetables are magic bullets. However, a primary factor in developing both heart disease and cancer is excess levels of insulin. Since fruits and vegetables are low-density carbohydrates, it is very difficult to overconsume them, and hence difficult to overproduce insulin. Beta-carotene levels in the bloodstream are simply an indication of increased fruit and vegetable consumption. However, when beta-carotene is given as a supplement in high doses, there is either no benefit or in some cases an actual increase in cancer.

How many servings of fruits and vegetables are Americans currently eating?

The goal set by the U.S. government is to eat five servings per day of fruits and vegetables. However, it is estimated that only a small percentage of Americans are meeting even that modest goal. Following the Soy Zone Diet, you would be eating ten to fifteen servings of fruits and vegetables per day. This represents two to three times the amounts recommended by the government. At this level of fruit and vegetable consumption, both heart disease and cancer are dramatically reduced.

What's the difference between eating fruits and drinking fruit juices?

Fruit juices are very concentrated sources of carbohydrates, without any fiber to slow their entry into the bloodstream. People rarely eat more than one piece of fresh fruit at a sitting, but can easily consume the equivalent of four to six pieces of fruit when drinking fruit juice. That amount of carbohydrate can cause a tremendous stimulation of insulin. It makes more hormonal sense to have an orange rather than a glass of orange juice.

What are the best carbohydrate sources of vitamins and minerals?

Exactly what your grandmother told you—fruits and vegetables. When fruits and vegetables are compared to grains and starches for their vitamin and mineral content *per gram* of carbohydrate, it quickly becomes evident that they are the true vitamin and mineral powerhouses. This is why vegetables and fruits are staples of the Soy Zone Diet and grains and starches are used in moderation. Vegetables and fruits provide the least amount of insulin stimulation while supplying more than adequate amounts of vitamins and minerals.

FATS

Does fat really make you fat?

Not really. It's actually excess insulin that makes you fat and keeps you fat. Insulin is a storage hormone. One of the consequences of excess insulin is that it increases the storage of incoming calories as fat and also prevents the release of stored fat for energy. In reality, dietary fat has no effect on insulin, whereas excess carbohydrate consumption has a significant impact on insulin secretion. To prevent excess insulin secretion, most of your carbohydrate should come from low-density sources, such as vegetables and fruits. Go easy on the high-density sources such as pasta, bagels, and starches.

Does this mean I can eat whatever fat I want?

No. You need to be selective about the kinds of fat you eat because all fats are not created equal. Fats are characterized by how much saturation (or solidity) they have. Isolated oils containing saturated fats are solid at room temperature. Most saturated fats are found in animal sources of protein. Unfortunately, saturated fats induce the body to make more cholesterol, thus increasing the likelihood of heart disease.

Monounsaturated fats are liquid at room temperature but get cloudy in the refrigerator. These are the healthiest kinds of fats because they have no adverse effect on cholesterol levels. Typical sources of monounsaturated fats include olives, avocado, and selected nuts, such as almonds, pistachios, and macadamia.

Finally, there are polyunsaturated fats. These fats typically come from oil seeds, such as soybean, flax, sunflower, and safflower. These fats aren't as heart-damaging as saturated fats, but they aren't as healthful as monounsaturated fats because of the adverse effects that Omega-6 fatty acids can have. Polyunsaturated fats that have been chemically transformed to make them solid (like margarine) contain heart-damaging trans fatty acids, which may increase your heart disease risk as much as saturated fat.

What are essential fatty acids?

Essential fatty acids are the building blocks for a group of hormones known as eicosanoids. There are two distinct groups of essential fatty acids, known as Omega-6 and Omega-3 fatty acids. However, only the long-chain essential fatty acids can be made into eicosanoids. Depending on the type of long-chain essential fatty acid, eicosanoids of very different and often opposite physiological functions will be made. Long-chain Omega-3 fatty acids (found in fish oil and algae oil supplements) make "good" eicosanoids and lead to improved cardiovascular, immune, and mental function. Long-chain Omega-6 fats, on the other hand, can lead to the excess production of "bad" eicosanoids, which can lead to heart disease and cancer.

This is why I recommend adding monounsaturated fats (which are poor in Omega-6 fats) to Soy Zone meals, and then supplementing the diet with sources (fish or fish and algae oils) rich in long-chain Omega-3 fatty acids. The supplementation decreases the ration of Omega-6 to Omega-3 fatty acids and dramatically improves your overall health. The correlation was clearly demonstrated in the recent four-year Lyon Heart Study showing a 65 percent reduction in fatal attacks primarily achieved by increasing your Omega-3 fatty acid intake and simultaneously decreasing your Omega-6 intake.

Is flax oil sufficient to meet long-chain Omega-3 fatty acid needs?

Flax oil is the richest source of short-chain Omega-3 fatty acids. However, supplementation with flax oil will probably not generate the optimal amounts of longer-chain Omega-3 fatty acids that your body requires. The body's ability to make long-chain Omega-3 fats, such as eicosapentaenoic acid (EPA) and docosahexaenoic acid (DHA), from short-chain Omega-3 fatty acids is limited. This is why vegetarians always have lower levels of EPA and DHA in their blood than non-vegetarians do. If you plan to use flaxseed oil as a source of short-chain Omega-3 fatty acids, then take no more than 1 tablespoon (15 grams) per day, and simultaneously try to remove as much Omega-6 fatty acid from your diet as possible to increase the Omega-3/Omega-6 fatty acid ratio.

13

World Health Implications for the Soy Zone Diet

Throughout this book, I've talked about the Soy Zone Diet as being the latest evolution of the Zone Diet. The fact is, the Zone is a diet that evolved from our earliest eating habits, when we first arrived on this planet some 100,000 years ago. We began as meat eaters consuming large amounts of low-fat animal protein as well as fruits and vegetables. We then switched to grains after we began farming, and now we find that the cheapest—and most environmentally friendly—form of protein lies in the simple soybean. I want to discuss briefly where we came from before I tell you where we're going.

In our relatively short time on this planet, we've come to dominate the 30 million species of life and to command the vast bulk of the earth's resources. In our early days of relentless expansion, we developed into formidable predators who caused the virtual extinction of all big-game species on the planet. In fact, it is estimated that neo-Paleolithic man consumed more than 200 to 300 grams of protein per day. As our meat supplies diminished, we were forced to become farmers some 10,000 years ago. The switch to agriculture caused significant protein malnutrition as we came to rely more and more on grains. At least, though, grains provided enough calories to survive.

During the last century, Americans' demand for animal protein has risen again. We have become a meat-eating culture, and we pushed our agricultural resources to the extreme in order to grow grains to feed the animals that we were feasting on. As a result, our natural resources have been diminishing at a frightening rate, which has been devastating to our environment.

Furthermore, many of the animals that we rely on for protein are now struggling for survival. For example, the world's population of fish has dropped dramatically, yet we need fish to supply long-chain Omega-3 fatty acids, which are critical for optimal brain function. Yet at the same time, many of us need to consume more protein if we want to improve our health.

Of all societies, the hunter-gatherer societies that existed prior to the advent of agriculture were the least environmentally exploitative of all human cultures. This is because hunter-gatherer societies worked in very close harmony with the ecosystem (with the exception of the over-consumption of big-game animals). Obviously, we can't go back to a hunter-gatherer culture with some 6 billion people on the face of the earth. But we do need to consider world health implications when a projected 9 billion people compete for the same limited resources by the year 2050. Actually, we don't have to look that far into the future. Billions of people today are suffering from protein malnutrition, and thus are at great risk for infectious disease.

The solution? We must change the type of protein we eat to conserve our dwindling natural resources without having to sacrifice our consumption of adequate levels of protein. Soy protein fits the bill.

An almost immediate improvement in world health would result simply by adding more soy protein to the diets of people who are protein-malnourished. Without adequate protein, these people have depressed immune systems that are incapable of fighting off the life-threatening infectious diseases that run rampant in underdeveloped countries. Simply adding isolated protein power to a bowl of high-density carbohydrates (like rice, millet, or corn) would improve the immune function of billions of people (and especially their children) within weeks. Just a few weeks on the Soy Zone Diet could improve the health status of much of the world. It seems almost too good to be true, but the hormones generated by the food we eat can work that fast.

To limit the strain put on our natural resources by increasing our consumption of animals, the only choice for a massive increase in protein production must come from plants. The only logical plant choice, of course, is the soybean. There is no known plant that has as much protein per gram of raw material as the soybean. Furthermore, the technology exists not only to isolate soy protein, but also to keep it in a form (i.e., dehydrated powders) that requires no refrigeration and has a virtually unlimited shelf life. These powders can be mixed into just about every type of food, and the technology exists to convert these powders into meat substitutes of all kinds.

With obesity on the rise in America, we actually have a different problem: We have too much food to eat, and our farmers continuously produce food surpluses (mostly grains). As a result of this surplus, we have the cheapest food on earth, and thus we consequently eat more of it than we need. Gluttony has always been one of the seven deadly sins, and the primary hormonal result of carbohydrate gluttony is excess insulin production, which is the greatest threat to our health care system.

Virtually every chronic "Western" disease is a direct or indirect consequence of excess insulin production. Unlike the underdeveloped world, Americans are getting adequate protein, so we can fight infectious disease more effectively. At the same time, though, we consume too many carbohydrates in the form of cheap and abundant breads, cereals, potatoes, rice, and pasta. Replacing many of these high-density carbohydrates with lower-density carbohydrates, such as vegetables and fruits, would dramatically reduce insulin levels, while simultaneously increasing vitamin and mineral intakes. In addition, replacing our intake of animal protein with soy protein could also have a dramatic effect on reducing our excess insulin levels, thereby increasing our ability to maintain insulin levels within the Zone where optimal health exists.

As you can see, we have a global paradox on our hands: Protein malnutrition is rampant in underdeveloped countries, and food gluttony (mostly excess carbohydrates) is rampant in industrialized countries. The Soy Zone Diet can provide the solution for everyone, since it provides a cheap, abundant form of protein without overtaxing our natural resources. I firmly believe this diet can enable billions of humans to live a better life in greater health and greater harmony with the world's environment.

In this book, I have tried to show how you can easily introduce a greater number of soy-based meals into your dietary lifestyle, and thus take an important step toward reaching your goal of a longer and healthier life. I want you to know, however, that being on the Soy Zone Diet is not an all-or-nothing proposition. Nutrition activists often demand that you totally revamp your diet if you want to experience any improved health benefits. Frankly, I am a little more realistic about lifestyle changes and think it's wise to proceed slowly. Give yourself at least a year to integrate the full Soy Zone Diet into your daily routine. The first step is to increase your consumption of soy protein and decrease your consumption of bread, crackers, and other starches. You can, of course, gain the maximum benefits by following all the rules of the Soy Zone.

My recommendation is simply to include more and more Soy Zone meals in your diet at a pace that you are comfortable with. Keep in mind that all of your other meals should still be based on the basic Zone principles of balance and moderation.

Finally, I leave you with the question that I posed in Chapter 1: "Do you want to live a longer and healthier life?" If the answer is yes, then you need to enter the Zone. The Soy Zone Diet is the healthiest version of the Zone Diet and causes the least disruption to our environment. If you want to be an activist for a better planet, then it is time to stand up and be counted. A good start would be to incorporate the Soy Zone Diet into your daily eating routine. The fact is, you're not faced with a hard choice if you want to live a longer life and help preserve the Earth's future.

Appendix A

Technical Support

I hope you now realize that the Soy Zone Diet may be the most powerful "drug" for improving daily performance (both mental and physical), for losing excess body fat, and for living a longer and healthier life. Although I use the phrase Soy Zone Diet, this is not a short-term program as much as a lifelong food management system. This system will give you better health through enhanced hormonal control, using the foods you already enjoy eating.

This is the seventh book I have written about the Zone technology. My first book, *The Zone,* was written primarily for cardiovascular physicians to alert them to the power that food has to alter hormone levels, specifically how the levels of the hormones insulin, glucagon, and eicosanoids vary with the macronutrient composition of each meal. However, *The Zone* is not the best introduction for a beginner to understand how simple the Zone technology is to follow. That's why I strongly recommend reading my recently published *A Week in the Zone* as a great introduction to Zone basics—plus *Zone-Perfect Meals in Minutes* and *Mastering the Zone* as more detailed "how-to" books for using the Zone Diet. Once you understand basic Zone logic, then you can refer back to *The Zone* to better understand the biochemistry behind it. And if you really want to learn how to reverse aging and extend your life, then I strongly recommend reading *The Anti-Aging Zone*. This is my manifesto of the entire Zone technology that I've developed. Although *The Anti-Aging Zone* is more complex than *The*

Zone, it provides the information and motivation to make the Zone Diet your lifelong ally to increase and enhance your longevity by reversing the aging process.

Although each of my books represents the latest research on the complex relationship between diet and hormonal response available at the time each book was written, the field is constantly changing. You can access the latest information on my dietary program from my website, www.drsears.com, which discusses my latest thoughts on this constantly evolving program. In addition, I continually update my site with new recipes (many of them vegetarian), new research information, and simple tips to make the Zone Diet incredibly easy to follow on a lifelong basis.

The mission of my web site is to serve as a clearinghouse for information not only about the Zone Diet but also about the latest research concerning how diet can affect various hormones and how these hormones have an impact on your longevity. Since this information is rapidly evolving, www.drsears.com should be your primary Internet destination to help you understand new research findings that I present to you in a digestible form (no pun intended).

Also consider www.drsears.com as your personal cyberspace resource to understand and easily integrate the lifestyle steps necessary for a longer and better life. If you would like to receive additional useful information showing you how simple and easy Zone living can be, please call this toll-free number: 1-800-404-8171.

Zone Validation Studies

Throughout this book, I have constantly stressed that the Zone Diet will lower insulin levels. I'm not just presenting a scientific theory. My statement is backed up by several well-regarded research studies that have been published over the last few years. These studies have strongly validated the concept of the Zone Diet: You can lower your insulin levels if you balance the amount of carbohydrates you eat with your amount of protein (which usually means decreasing your intake of carbohydrates while increasing your intake of protein).

The first data validating the Zone Diet appeared in 1998 in two separate studies involving Type 2 diabetics. (About 90 percent of diabetics have the Type 2 kind, which means their bodies make too much insulin because their cells need large amounts in order to respond to the hormone.) As a result of having too much insulin, Type 2 diabetics are more likely to have heart attacks, strokes, amputations, blindness, and impotence than the general population. More important, they die five to ten years earlier than the general population.

Type 2 diabetics are thus the ideal subjects to determine whether or not a diet based on balancing protein and carbohydrate can lower insulin levels. The following table shows data from the study I conducted for an HMO with Type 2 diabetics, looking at the most important blood parameters after following a Zone Diet for six weeks.

Type 2 Diabetic Study (n=68)			
Parameter	**Start**	**6 Weeks**	**% Change**
Insulin	28	21	-23
Triglycerides	189	162	-14
HDL Cholesterol	45	49	+8
TG/HDL	4.2	3.1	-26

These people were instructed to follow a Zone Diet after having spent the previous year following the American Diabetes Association diet (which includes more high-density carbohydrates, such as grains and starches). The drop of elevated insulin in these patients after only six weeks represents a major step toward reducing their likelihood of heart attack. Likewise, there was a drop in triglycerides, a corresponding rise in HDL cholesterol, and, most important, a reduction in the triglyceride-to-HDL cholesterol (TG/HDL) ratio, which—according to a Harvard Medical School study—is also an exceptionally powerful predictor of a decreased likelihood of heart attacks. From the study in the table above you can see that the drop in the triglyceride-to-HDL cholesterol ratio was almost exactly equal to the drop in insulin levels. This supports my contention that the triglyceride-to-HDL cholesterol ratio is a good surrogate marker for insulin.

The power of science relies upon confirmation of results by other independent investigators. In other words, can someone else do an experiment similar to the one that I did and get essentially the same result? It turns out that my study was confirmed in 1998 by a group of Australian investigators. The only difference was that they took their patients' first blood samples after only three days on the Zone Diet, as opposed to the six weeks in my study. Amazingly, the insulin levels in their Type 2 patients were reduced by 36 percent by following the Zone Diet for just three days. In fact, overweight patients without Type 2 diabetes saw their insulin levels drop by 40 percent in the first three days following the same diet. There are very few drugs that can act that fast.

Is it possible that these changes in insulin levels could occur even faster, like after a single meal? That was the question posed by several Harvard Medical School investigators in 1999. In this study, they fed overweight adolescent boys three types of vegetarian meals. Two of the meals consisted of oatmeal, with the only difference being that one meal consisted of instant oatmeal flavored with glucose, and the other consisted of steel-cut oats flavored with fructose. The balance of protein to carbohydrate, the same in both of these meals, was about 0.3 (far below the lowest limits of the Zone). The third meal was a Zone meal (with a protein-to-carbohydrate ratio of 0.8) consisting of an omelet containing low-fat cheese, spinach, and tomato. In addition, they also ate half a grapefruit and some apple slices. (As much as I like oatmeal, the vegetarian Zone meal used in the study sure sounds a lot more appetizing to me.) All three meals contained the same number of calories.

The researchers at Harvard Medical School found that even this single meal had an effect on insulin levels. After eating the Zone meal, the boys had significantly lower levels of insulin secretion compared to when they ate the other two non-Zone meals. Even more striking than the difference in insulin secretion was the difference in their secretion of the hormone glucagon. (Remember that glucagon is the hormone stimulated by protein in the diet, and it's responsible for maintaining steady blood sugar levels.) In the two non-Zone meals, glucagon levels were depressed for the next five hours after the meal. On the other hand, glucagon levels were elevated on the Zone meal and didn't drop down to their starting levels until five hours later (which is why you need to eat every five hours on the Soy Zone Diet). Therefore, only with the Zone meal was a favorable balance of insulin and glucagon achieved to maintain more stable blood sugar levels to the brain. Not surprisingly, after eating a Zone meal, the young boys consumed less food at their next meal compared to the amounts they ate following non-Zone meals—even though the meals all had the same number of calories. As the investigators stated:

> These results demonstrate that commonly consumed meals containing identical amounts of energy may have markedly dif-

ferent effects on metabolism, perceived hunger, and subsequent food intake.

Translated into non-Harvardese, they are saying that a calorie is *not* a calorie when it comes to hormonal and metabolic responses. What is important is the balance of protein to carbohydrate, because that balance will control the hormonal responses of insulin and glucagon for the next four to six hours. This is the kind of clinical result that makes the traditional nutritional community very nervous, because it calls into question their constant mantra that a calorie is a calorie, and therefore weight gain and weight loss are simply a matter of counting calories regardless of what food source they come from. In fact, the more you learn about the hormonal effect of food, the more you'll see that virtually every nutritional dogma that nutritionists have espoused over the years as to what constitutes a healthy diet becomes suspect.

Additional supporting evidence for that statement comes from a recent 1999 study published in the *International Journal of Obesity* in which overweight patients were put on two different diets. Both of the diets contained the same number of calories and the same amount of fat (about 30 percent of total calories). The only difference was the protein-to-carbohydrate ratio. One diet was a high-carbohydrate diet (a protein-to-carbohydrate ratio of 0.2), and the other diet was a Zone diet (a protein-to-carbohydrate ratio of 0.6). Those patients following the Zone diet lost almost twice as much body fat as those patients following the high-carbohydrate diet. If a calorie is a calorie, then it is hard to explain these results. However, if you are thinking hormonally (i.e., fat loss is accomplished by lowering elevated insulin levels), the results are easy to understand.

As impressive as these Zone validation studies are, the results would have been even better had soy protein replaced much of the animal protein. This is because the soy protein would have had a far greater insulin-lowering effect.

Calculation of Lean Body Mass

A rapid way to determine your lean body mass is simply to use a tape measure and scale. You should make all measurements on bare skin (not through clothing), and make sure that the tape fits snugly but does not compress the skin and underlying tissue. Take all measurements three times and calculate the average. All measurements should be in inches.

CALCULATING BODY-FAT PERCENTAGES FOR FEMALES

There are five steps you must take to calculate your percentage of body fat:

1. While keeping the tape level, measure your hips at their widest point, and your waist at the umbilicus (i.e., belly button). It is critical that you measure at the belly button and not at the narrowest point of your waist. Take each of these measurements three times and compute the average.

2. Measure your height in inches without shoes.

3. Record your height, waist, and hip measurements on the accompanying worksheet.

4. Find each of these measurements in the appropriate column in the accompanying tables and record the constants on the worksheet.

5. Add constants A and B, then subtract constant C for this sum and round to the nearest whole number. That figure is your percentage of body fat.

Worksheet for Women to Calculate Their Percentage of Body Fat

Average hip measurement _____ (used for Constant A)

Average abdomen measurement _____ (used for Constant B)

Height _____ (used for Constant C)

Using Table 1, look up each of the average measurements and your height in the appropriate column.

Constant A = _____

Constant B = _____

Constant C = _____

To determine your approximate percentage of body fat, then add Constant A and B. From that total, subtract Constant C. The result is your percentage of body fat.

Calculating Body-Fat Percentages for Men

There are four steps you must take to determine your body-fat percentage:

1. While keeping the tape level, measure the circumference of your waist at the umbilicus (i.e., belly button). Measure three times and compute the average.

2. Measure your wrist at the space between your dominant hand and your wrist bone, at the location where your wrist bends.

3. Record these measurements on the worksheet for males.

4. Subtract your wrist measurement from your waist measurement and find the resulting value listed in the table. On the left-hand side

of this table, find your weight. Proceed to right from your weight and down from your waist-minus-wrist measurement. Where these two points intersect, read your body fat percentage.

Worksheet for Men to Calculate Their Percentage of Body Fat

Average waist measurement _____ (inches)

Average wrist measurement _____ (inches)

Subtract the wrist measurement from the waist measurement. Use Table 2 to find your weight. Then find your "waist minus wrist" number. Where the two columns intersect is your approximate percentage of body fat.

Calculating Lean Body Mass for Both Females and Males

Now that you know your body-fat percentage, the next step is to use this figure to calculate the weight in pounds of the fat portion of your total body weight. (Note: If you are off either chart, assume you have 50 percent body fat.) This is done by multiplying your weight by your percentage of body fat (Remember to use a decimal point—15 percent is 0.15 for example).

(Weight) x (% of body fat) = total body-fat weight

Once you know the weight of your total body fat, you subtract that total fat weight from your total weight, which results in your lean body mass. Lean body mass is the total weight of all nonfat body tissue.

_____ Your total weight

- _____ Your total of body fat

= _____ Your lean body mass

Lean body mass = total weight - total body-fat weight

Table 1

Conversion Constants for Prediction
of Percentage of Body Fat in Females

Hips		Abdomen		Height	
Inches	Constant A	Inches	Constant B	Inches	Constant C
30	33.48	20	14.22	55	33.52
30.5	33.83	20.5	14.40	55.5	33.67
31	34.87	21.0	14.93	56	34.13
31.5	35.22	21.5	15.11	56.5	34.28
32	36.27	22	15.64	57	34.74
32.5	36.62	22.5	15.82	57.5	34.89
33	37.67	23	16.35	58	35.35
33.5	38.02	23.5	16.53	58.5	35.50
34	39.06	24	17.06	59	35.96
34.5	39.41	24.5	17.24	59.5	36.11
35	40.46	25	17.78	60	36.57
35.5	40.81	25.5	17.96	60.5	36.72
36	41.86	26	18.49	61	37.18
36.5	42.21	26.5	18.67	61.5	37.33
37	43.25	27	19.20	62	37.79
37.5	43.60	27.5	19.38	62.5	37.94
38	44.65	28	19.91	63	38.40
38.5	45.32	28.5	20.27	63.5	38.70
39	46.05	29	20.62	64	39.01
39.5	46.40	29.5	20.80	64.5	39.16
40	47.44	30	21.33	65	39.62
40.5	47.79	30.5	21.51	65.5	39.77
41	48.84	31	22.04	66	40.23
41.5	49.19	31.5	22.22	66.5	40.38
42	50.24	32	22.75	67	40.84
42.5	50.59	32.5	22.93	67.5	40.99
43	51.64	33	23.46	68	41.45
43.5	51.99	33.5	23.64	68.5	41.60
44	53.03	34	24.18	69	42.06
44.5	53.41	34.5	24.36	69.5	42.21

Hips		Abdomen		Height	
Inches	Constant A	Inches	Constant B	Inches	Constant C
45	54.53	35	24.89	70	42.67
45.5	54.86	35.5	25.07	70.5	42.82
46	55.83	36	25.60	71	43.28
46.5	56.18	36.5	25.78	71.5	43.43
47	57.22	37	26.31	72	43.89
47.5	57.57	37.5	26.49	72.5	44.04
48	58.62	38	27.02	73	44.50
48.5	58.97	38.5	27.20	73.5	44.65
49	60.02	39	27.73	74	45.11
49.5	60.37	39.5	27.91	74.5	45.26
50	61.42	40	28.44	75	45.72
50.5	61.77	40.5	28.62	75.5	45.87
51	62.81	41	29.15	76	46.32
51.5	63.16	41.5	29.33		
52	64.21	42	29.87		
52.5	64.56	42.5	30.05		
53	65.61	43	30.58		
53.5	65.96	43.5	30.76		
54	67.00	44	31.29		
54.5	67.35	44.5	31.47		
55	68.40	45	32.00		
55.5	68.75	45.5	32.18		
56	69.80	46	32.71		
56.5	70.15	46.5	32.89		
57	71.19	47	33.42		
57.5	71.54	47.5	33.60		
58	72.59	48	34.13		
58.5	72.94	48.5	34.31		
59	73.99	49	34.84		
59.5	74.34	49.5	35.02		
60	75.39	50	35.56		

Table 2

Male Percentage Body Fat Calculations

Waist-Wrist (in inches)	22	22.5	23	23.5	24
Weight (in lbs.)					
120	4	6	8	10	12
125	4	6	7	9	11
130	3	5	7	9	11
135	3	5	7	8	10
140	3	5	6	8	10
145		4	6	7	9
150		4	6	7	9
155		4	5	6	8
160		4	5	6	8
165		3	5	6	8
170		3	4	6	7
175			4	6	7
180			4	5	7
185			4	5	6
190			4	5	6
195			3	5	6
200			3	4	6
205				4	5
210				4	5
215				4	5
220				4	5
225				3	4
230				3	4
235				3	4
240					4
245					4
250					4
255					3
260					3
265					
270					
275					
280					
285					
290					
295					
300					

24.5	25	25.5	26	26.5	27	27.5
14	16	18	20	21	23	25
13	15	17	19	20	22	24
12	14	16	18	20	21	23
12	13	15	17	19	20	22
11	13	15	16	18	19	21
11	12	14	15	17	19	20
10	12	13	15	16	18	19
10	11	13	14	16	17	19
9	11	12	14	15	17	18
9	10	12	13	15	16	17
9	10	11	13	14	15	17
8	10	11	12	12	15	16
8	9	10	12	13	14	16
8	9	10	11	13	14	15
7	8	10	11	12	13	15
7	8	9	11	12	13	14
7	8	9	10	11	12	14
6	8	9	10	11	12	13
6	7	8	9	11	12	13
6	7	8	9	10	11	12
6	7	8	9	10	11	12
6	7	8	9	10	11	12
5	6	7	8	9	10	11
5	6	7	8	9	10	11
5	6	7	8	9	10	11
5	6	7	8	9	9	10
5	6	6	7	8	9	10
4	5	6	7	8	9	10
4	5	6	7	8	9	10
4	5	6	7	8	8	9
4	5	6	7	7	8	9
4	5	5	6	7	8	9
4	4	5	6	7	8	9
4	4	5	6	7	8	8
3	4	5	6	7	7	8
3	4	5	6	6	7	8
3	4	5	5	6	7	8

Waist-Wrist (in inches)	28	28.5	29	29.5	30	30.5	31
Weight (in lbs.)							
120	27	29	31	33	35	37	39
125	26	28	30	32	33	35	37
130	25	27	28	30	32	34	36
135	24	26	27	29	31	32	34
140	23	24	26	28	29	31	33
145	22	23	25	27	28	30	31
150	21	23	24	26	27	29	30
155	20	22	23	25	26	28	29
160	19	21	22	24	25	27	28
165	19	20	22	23	24	26	27
170	18	19	21	22	24	25	26
175	17	19	20	21	23	24	25
180	17	18	19	21	22	23	25
185	16	18	19	20	21	23	24
190	16	17	18	19	21	22	23
195	15	16	18	19	20	21	22
200	15	16	17	18	19	21	22
205	14	15	17	18	19	20	21
210	14	15	16	17	18	19	21
215	13	15	16	17	18	19	20
220	13	14	15	16	17	18	19
225	13	14	15	16	17	18	19
230	12	13	14	15	16	17	18
235	12	13	14	15	16	17	18
240	12	13	14	15	16	17	17
245	11	12	13	14	15	16	17
250	11	12	13	14	15	16	17
255	11	12	13	14	14	15	16
260	10	11	12	13	14	15	16
265	10	11	12	13	14	15	15
270	10	11	12	13	13	14	15
275	10	11	11	12	13	14	15
280	9	10	11	12	13	14	14
285	9	10	11	12	12	13	14
290	9	10	11	11	12	13	14
295	9	10	10	11	12	13	14
300	9	9	10	11	12	12	13

31.5	32	32.5	33	33.5	34	34.5
41	43	45	47	49	50	52
39	41	43	45	46	48	50
37	39	41	43	44	46	48
36	38	39	41	43	44	46
34	36	38	39	41	43	44
33	35	36	38	39	41	43
32	33	35	36	38	40	41
31	32	34	35	37	38	40
30	31	33	34	35	37	38
29	30	31	33	34	36	37
28	29	30	32	33	34	36
27	28	29	31	32	33	35
26	27	28	30	31	32	34
25	26	28	29	30	31	33
24	26	27	28	29	30	32
24	25	26	27	28	30	31
23	24	25	26	28	29	30
22	23	25	26	27	28	29
22	23	24	25	26	27	28
21	22	23	24	25	26	28
20	22	23	24	25	26	27
20	21	22	23	24	25	26
19	20	21	22	23	24	25
19	20	21	22	23	24	25
18	19	20	21	22	23	24
18	19	20	21	22	23	24
18	18	19	20	21	22	23
17	18	19	20	21	22	23
17	18	19	19	20	21	22
16	17	18	19	20	21	22
16	17	18	19	19	20	21
16	16	17	18	19	20	21
15	16	17	18	19	19	20
15	16	17	17	18	19	20
15	15	16	17	18	19	19
14	15	16	17	17	18	19
14	15	16	16	17	18	19

Waist-Wrist (in inches)	35	35.5	36	36.5	37
Weight (in lbs.)					
120	54				
125	52	54			
130	50	52	53	55	
135	48	50	51	53	55
140	46	48	49	51	53
145	44	46	47	49	51
150	43	44	46	47	49
155	41	43	44	46	47
160	40	41	43	44	46
165	38	40	41	43	44
170	37	39	40	41	43
175	36	37	39	40	41
180	35	36	37	39	40
185	34	35	36	38	39
190	33	34	35	37	38
195	32	33	34	35	37
200	31	32	33	35	36
205	30	31	32	34	35
210	29	30	32	33	34
215	29	30	31	32	33
220	28	29	30	31	32
225	27	28	29	30	31
230	26	27	28	30	31
235	26	27	28	29	30
240	25	26	27	28	29
245	25	26	27	27	28
250	24	25	26	27	28
255	24	24	25	26	27
260	23	24	25	26	27
265	22	23	24	25	26
270	22	23	24	25	25
275	22	22	23	24	25
280	21	22	23	24	24
285	21	21	22	23	24
290	20	21	22	23	23
295	20	21	21	22	23
300	19	20	21	22	22

37.5	38	38.5	39	39.5	40	40.5
54						
52	54	55				
50	52	53	55			
49	50	52	53	55		
47	48	50	51	53	54	
45	47	48	50	51	52	54
44	45	47	48	49	51	52
43	44	45	47	48	49	51
41	43	44	45	47	48	49
40	41	43	44	45	46	48
39	40	41	43	44	45	46
38	39	40	41	43	44	45
37	38	39	40	41	43	44
36	37	38	39	40	41	43
35	36	37	38	39	40	42
34	35	36	37	38	39	40
33	34	35	36	37	38	39
32	33	34	35	36	37	38
32	33	34	35	36	37	38
31	32	33	34	35	36	37
30	31	32	33	34	35	36
29	30	31	32	33	34	35
29	30	31	31	32	33	34
28	29	30	31	32	33	34
27	28	29	30	31	32	33
27	28	29	29	30	31	32
26	27	28	29	30	31	31
26	27	27	28	29	30	31
25	26	27	28	29	29	30
25	26	26	27	28	29	30
24	25	26	27	27	28	29
24	25	25	26	27	28	28
23	24	25	26	26	27	28

Waist-Wrist (in inches)	41	41.5	42	42.5	43	43.5
Weight (in lbs.)						
120						
125						
130						
135						
140						
145						
150						
155						
160						
165	55					
170	54	55				
175	52	53	55			
180	50	52	53	54		
185	49	50	51	53	54	55
190	48	49	50	51	52	54
195	46	47	49	50	51	52
200	45	46	47	48	50	51
205	44	45	46	47	48	49
210	43	44	45	46	47	48
215	42	43	44	45	46	47
220	41	42	43	44	45	46
225	40	41	42	43	44	45
230	39	40	41	42	44	44
235	38	39	40	41	42	43
240	37	38	39	40	41	42
245	36	37	38	39	40	41
250	35	36	37	38	39	40
255	34	35	36	37	38	39
260	34	35	35	36	37	38
265	33	34	35	36	36	37
270	32	33	34	35	36	37
275	32	32	33	34	35	36
280	31	32	33	33	34	35
285	30	31	32	33	34	34
290	30	31	31	32	33	34
295	29	30	31	32	32	33
300	29	29	30	31	32	33

44	44.5	45	45.5	46	46.5	47
55						
53	55					
52	53	54	55			
51	52	53	54	55		
49	50	51	53	54	55	
48	49	50	51	52	53	54
47	48	49	50	51	52	53
46	47	48	49	50	51	52
45	46	47	48	49	50	51
44	45	46	47	48	49	50
43	44	45	46	46	47	48
42	43	44	44	45	46	47
41	42	43	44	44	45	46
40	41	42	43	44	44	45
39	40	41	42	43	43	44
38	39	40	41	42	43	43
37	38	39	40	41	42	43
37	38	38	39	40	41	42
36	37	38	38	39	40	41
35	36	37	38	39	39	40
35	35	36	37	38	39	39
34	35	36	36	37	38	39
33	34	35	36	36	37	38

Waist-Wrist (in inches)	47.5	48	48.5	49	49.5	50
Weight (in lbs.)						
120						
125						
130						
135						
140						
145						
150						
155						
160						
165						
170						
175						
180						
185						
190						
195						
200						
205						
210						
215	55					
220	54	55				
225	53	54	55			
230	52	53	54	55		
235	51	51	52	53	54	55
240	49	50	51	52	53	54
245	48	49	50	51	52	53
250	47	48	49	50	51	52
255	46	47	48	49	50	51
260	45	46	47	48	49	50
265	44	45	46	47	48	49
270	43	44	45	46	47	48
275	43	43	44	45	46	47
280	42	43	43	44	45	46
285	41	42	43	43	44	45
290	40	41	42	43	43	44
295	39	40	41	42	43	43
300	39	39	40	41	42	43

Zone Food Blocks
for Making
Soy Zone Meals

Any long-term dietary program is simply an accounting system to keep track of the macronutrient balance. Many of these systems are based on counting calories, or fat grams, or carbohydrates. If you've followed a traditional diet plan, you know all too well that the amount of weight lost on these plans is limited primarily by a constant sense of deprivation. Once you go off your diet, your lost pounds soon return.

The Soy Zone Diet is based on a different concept—balance. You are trying to maintain a balance of protein to carbohydrate at each meal and snack to generate the appropriate hormonal response. If you get the right balance, you will lose excess body fat because you are lowering excess insulin, and you won't feel hungry between meals because you are maintaining constant blood sugar levels. In addition, you'll also live longer and have a lower risk of developing a chronic disease like heart disease, diabetes or cancer as long as you follow the Soy Zone Diet. This is because the Soy Zone Diet is not a diet, but a lifelong plan based on balance and moderation.

The Soy Zone Diet is like balancing your checkbook. In your checkbook, you keep track of money coming in and money going out. You don't have to be precise to the penny on your balance, but you do want to make sure you have enough money to write a check that won't bounce. The Soy Zone Diet is similar in that the better you balance the protein and carbohydrate at your last meal, the less likely you'll write a hormonal check that bounces. I believe the easiest way to balance your hormonal checkbook is by using the Zone Food Block method.

When you determine the amount of carbohydrate you plan to eat at a meal, remember that you only need to count those carbohydrates that stimulate insulin secretion. This means that you should subtract out the fiber content in any carbohydrate because fiber doesn't trigger the release of insulin. So if you're eating a bowl of oatmeal containing 27 grams of carbohydrates and 4 grams of fiber, you're only really getting 23 grams of carbohydrates. Don't worry, all of these calculations are done for you when you use the Zone Food Blocks.

On the flip side, you want to choose vegetable *protein* sources that are relatively low in fiber. This is because fiber prevents the absorption of protein. About 30 percent of the protein in vegetarian sources is not absorbed because it is packaged in the food's fiber. The lower the fiber content of a protein, the higher the percentage of protein that will be absorbed. Tofu, soy meat substitutes, and soy powder are all high-protein, low-fiber choices, which means that virtually all the protein will be absorbed.

Making Soy Zone Meals simply requires balancing the number of protein, carbohydrate, and fat block servings in equal proportions. The typical female will need three Zone Blocks *each* of protein, carbohydrate, and fat at every meal, whereas the typical male will need four Zone Blocks of *each* macronutrient at every meal. Zone snacks consist of one Zone Block of each of the three macronutrients.

Thus, for a typical female, each meal would consist of three Zone Protein Blocks, three Zone Carbohydrate Blocks, and three Zone Fat Blocks. For the typical male, each Soy Zone meal consists of four Zone Protein Blocks, four Zone Carbohydrate Blocks, and four Zone Fat Blocks. A snack is one Zone Protein Block, one Zone Carbohydrate block, and one Zone Fat block. Feel free to mix and match the Zone Food Blocks within each macronutrient group as long as they add up to your required numbers at the end of the meal.

Be aware, though, that many vegetarian protein sources tend to have both protein and carbohydrate blocks, so take this into account when constructing meals. Here is a listing of many popular foods broken down into Zone Protein, Carbohydrate, and Fat blocks. If you want a more complete list, my book *Zone Food Blocks* contains a listing of thousands of food items broken down into their Zone Food Blocks.

ZONE SOY PROTEIN BLOCKS (EACH PORTION CONTAINS APPROXIMATELY 7 GRAMS OF ABSORBABLE PROTEIN PER ZONE BLOCK)

Protein-Rich Soy Sources	per Zone Block
Protein powder	7 grams
Soybean hamburger crumbles	$^1/_3$ cup
Soybean Canadian bacon	3 slices
Soybean frozen sausage	1 link
Soybean hot dog	1 link
Tofu, firm and extra-firm	2–3 oz

MIXED PROTEIN SOURCES (THESE CONTAIN MORE CARBOHYDRATES—READ THE LABELS CAREFULLY)

	per Zone Block	Associated Carbohydrate Blocks
Soybeans, boiled	$^1/_4$ cup	$^2/_3$
Soy milk	8 oz	1
Soy flour	10 grams	1
Soybean hamburger	$^3/_4$ patty	$^1/_3$
Tempeh	$1^1/_2$ oz	1
Tofu, silken	5 oz	$^1/_2$
Tofu, soft	4 oz	$^1/_3$

ZONE CARBOHYDRATE BLOCKS (EACH PORTION CONTAINS APPROXIMATELY 9 GRAMS OF INSULIN-STIMULATING CARBOHYDRATES PER ZONE BLOCK)

FAVORABLE CARBOHYDRATES (USE PRIMARILY)

Cooked vegetables	per Zone Block
Artichoke	4 large
Artichoke hearts	1 cup
Asparagus	12 spears
Beans, green or wax	1^1/$_2$ cups
Beans, black	^{1}/$_4$ cup
Bok choy	3 cups
Broccoli	3 cups
Brussels sprouts	1^1/$_2$ cups
Cabbage (red or green)	3 cups
Cauliflower	4 cups
Chickpeas	^{1}/$_4$ cup
Collard greens, chopped	2 cups
Eggplant	1^1/$_2$ cups
Kale	2 cups
Kidney beans	^{1}/$_4$ cup
Leeks	1 cup
Lentils	^{1}/$_4$ cup
Mushrooms, whole, boiled	2 cups
Onions (all types), chopped, boiled	^{1}/$_2$ cup

Okra, sliced	1 cup
Sauerkraut	1 cup
Squash, yellow, sliced and boiled	2 cups
Spinach	$3^1/_2$ cups
Swiss chard	$2^1/_2$ cups
Tomato, canned, chopped	1 cup
Tomato, puree	$^1/_2$ cup
Tomato sauce	$^1/_2$ cup
Turnip, mashed	$1^1/_2$ cups
Turnip greens, chopped, boiled	4 cups
Zucchini	2 cups

Raw vegetables	**per block**
Alfalfa sprouts	10 cups
Bamboo shoots	4 cups
Bean sprouts	3 cups
Beans, green	2 cups
Bell peppers (green or red)	2
Broccoli	4 cups
Brussels sprouts	$1^1/_2$ cups
Cabbage, shredded	4 cups
Cauliflower	4 cups
Celery, sliced	2 cups
Chickpeas	$^1/_4$ cup

Cucumber (medium)	$1^1/_2$
Endive, chopped	10 cups
Escarole, chopped	10 cups
Jalapeño peppers	2 cups
Lettuce, iceberg	2 heads
Lettuce, romaine, shredded	10 cups
Mushrooms, chopped	4 cups
Onion, chopped	$1^1/_2$ cups
Radishes, sliced	4 cups
Scallions	3 cups
Shallots, diced	$1^1/_2$ cups
Snow peas	$1^1/_2$ cups
Spinach, chopped	20 cups
Tomato	2
Tomato, cherry	2 cups
Tomato, chopped	$1^1/_2$ cups
Water chestnuts	$1/_3$ cup
Watercress	10 cups
Fruits (fresh, frozen, or canned light)	**per block**
Apple	$1/_2$
Applesauce (unsweetened)	$1/_3$ cup
Apricots	3

Blackberries	3/4 cup
Blueberries	1/2 cup
Boysenberries	1/2 cup
Cherries	8
Fruit cocktail, canned in water	1/3 cup
Grapes	1/2 cup
Grapefruit	1/2
Kiwi	1
Nectarine	1/2
Orange	1/2
Orange, mandarin, canned in water	1/3 cup
Peach	1
Peaches, canned in water	1/2 cup
Pear	1/2
Pineapple, cubed	1/2 cup
Plum	1
Raspberries	1 cup
Strawberries, diced fine	1 cup

Grains	**per block**
Barley, dry	1/2 tablespoon
Oatmeal, dry (slow cooking)	1/2 oz
Oatmeal, cooked (slow cooking)	1/3 cup

UNFAVORABLE CARBOHYDRATES (USE IN MODERATION)

Cooked vegetables	per block
Acorn squash	1/2 cup
Beans, baked	1/4 cup
Beans, refried	1/4 cup
Beets, sliced	1/2 cup
Butternut squash	1/2 cup
Carrots, sliced	1 cup
Corn	1/4 cup
French fries	5 pieces
Lima beans	1/4 cup
Parsnip	1/3 cup
Peas	1/2 cup
Pinto beans	1/4 cup
Potato, baked	1/4
Potato, boiled	1/3 cup
Potato, mashed	1/4 cup
Sweet potato, baked	1/3 cup

Fruits	per block
Banana	1/3
Cantaloupe	1/4 melon
Cranberries	3/4 cup
Cranberry sauce	3 teaspoons
Dates	2 pieces

Guava	$^1/_2$ cup
Honeydew melon, cubed	$^2/_3$ cup
Kumquat	3 pieces
Mango, sliced	$^1/_3$ cup
Papaya, cubed	$^3/_4$ cup
Pineapple, diced	$^1/_2$ cup
Prunes, dried	2
Raisins	1 tablespoon
Watermelon, diced	$^3/_4$ cup

Fruit juices	**per block**
Apple juice	$^1/_3$ cup
Apple cider	$^1/_3$ cup
Cranberry juice	$^1/_4$ cup
Fruit punch	$^1/_4$ cup
Grape juice	$^1/_4$ cup
Grapefruit juice	$^1/_3$ cup
Lemon juice	$^1/_3$ cup
Lemonade, unsweetened	$^1/_3$ cup
Lime juice	$^1/_3$ cup
Orange juice	$^1/_3$ cup
Pineapple juice	$^1/_4$ cup
Tomato juice	1 cup
Vegetable juice	$^3/_4$ cup

Grains and breads	per block
Bagel (small)	$1/4$
Biscuit	$1/2$
Bread crumbs	$1/2$ oz
Bread, whole-grain	$1/2$ slice
Bread, white	$1/2$ slice
Breadstick, hard	1 small
Breadstick, soft	$1/2$ piece
Buckwheat, dry	$1/2$ oz
Bulgar wheat, dry	$1/2$ oz
Cereal, breakfast	$1/2$ oz
Cornbread	1-square-inch piece
Cornstarch	4 teaspoons
Couscous, dry	$1/2$ oz
Cracker, graham	$1 1/2$
Cracker, saltine	4
Cracker, Triscuit	3
Croissant, plain	$1/4$
Crouton	$1/2$ oz
Donut, plain	$1/3$
English muffin	$1/4$
Granola	$1/2$ oz
Grits, cooked	$1/3$ cup
Melba toast	$1/2$ oz

Millet, dry	$^1/_2$ oz
Muffin, blueberry (mini)	$^1/_2$
Noodles, egg (cooked)	$^1/_4$ cup
Pancake (4")	1
Pasta, cooked	$^1/_4$ cup
Pita bread	$^1/_4$ pocket
Pita bread, mini	$^1/_2$ pocket
Popcorn, popped	2 cups
Rice, brown (cooked)	$^1/_5$ cup
Rice, long-grain (cooked)	$^1/_3$ cup
Rice, white (cooked)	$^1/_5$ cup
Rice cake	1
Roll, bulky	$^1/_4$
Roll, dinner (small)	$^1/_2$
Roll, hamburger	$^1/_2$
Taco shell	1
Tortilla, corn (6")	1
Tortilla, flour (8")	$^1/_2$
Waffle	$^1/_2$

Others	**per block**
Barbecue sauce	2 tablespoons
Cake (small slice)	$^1/_3$
Candy bar	$^1/_4$

Catsup	2 tablespoons
Cocktail sauce	2 tablespoons
Cookie (small)	1
Honey	$1/2$ tablespoon
Ice cream, regular	$1/4$ cup
Ice cream, premium	$1/5$ cup
Jam or jelly	2 tablespoons
Plum sauce	$1 1/2$ tablespoons
Molasses, light	$1/2$ tablespoon
Potato chips	$1/2$ oz
Pretzels	$1/2$ oz
Relish, pickle	4 teaspoons
Salsa	$1/2$ cup
Sugar, brown	2 teaspoons
Sugar, granulated	2 teaspoons
Sugar, confectioners'	1 tablespoon
Syrup, maple	2 teaspoons
Syrup, pancake	2 teaspoons
Teriyaki sauce	1 tablespoon
Tortilla chips	$1/2$ oz
Alcohol	**per block**
Beer, light	6 oz
Beer, regular	4 oz

Distilled spirits	1 oz
Wine (red or white)	4 oz

FAT SOURCES (APPROXIMATELY 3 GRAMS FAT PER ZONE BLOCK)

Best (rich in monounsaturated fats)	per block
Almonds	3
Almond oil	$2/3$ teaspoon
Avocado	1 tablespoon
Canola oil	$2/3$ teaspoon
Cashews	3
Guacamole	2 tablespoons
Macadamia nuts	2
Olives, black (medium)	5
Olive oil	$2/3$ teaspoon
Peanuts	6
Peanut oil	$2/3$ teaspoon
Peanut butter, natural	1 teaspoon
Pistachios	3
Sesame oil	$2/3$ teaspoon
Tahini	$1/3$ tablespoon

Appendix E

Synthesis of DHA

Throughout the book, I have emphasized the need to supplement your diet with long-chain Omega-3 fatty acids such as docosahexaenoic acid (DHA). Once you see how hard it is for your body to manufacture DHA from the foods you eat, you'll see why supplementation is so important. Although DHA can be synthesized from the short-chain Omega-3 fatty acid alpha-linolenic acid (ALA), found in many plants, the rate is excruciatingly slow and generates only low concentrations of these critical long-chain Omega-3 fatty acids. Theoretically, if you consume enough ALA, you should make more than adequate amounts of DHA. Unfortunately, it is not as easy as that, as shown in the figure below.

Synthesis of DHA from ALA (found in linseed oil, flaxseed oil, and other plant oils)

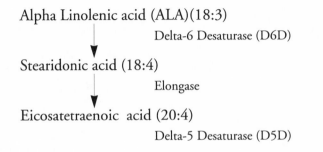

Alpha Linolenic acid (ALA)(18:3)

Delta-6 Desaturase (D6D)

Stearidonic acid (18:4)

Elongase

Eicosatetraenoic acid (20:4)

Delta-5 Desaturase (D5D)

Eicosapentanoic acid (EPA) (20:5)

       ↓   Elongase

Docosapentaenoic acid (22:5)

       ↓   Elongase

Tetrapentaenoic acid (24:5)

       ↓   Delta-6 Desaturase (D6D)

Tetrahexaenoic acid (24:6)

       ↓   Peroxisome beta oxidation

Docosahexanenoic acid (DHA) (22:6)

       ↓   Peroxisome beta oxidation

Eicosapentanoic acid (EPA) (20:5)

The reason why I outline this exceptionally complicated biochemical pathway is to demonstrate that it's not easy for humans to *make* DHA, whereas eating DHA in the form of supplements is easy. In fact, consuming preformed DHA is like taking a short trip to the beach in Santa Monica from downtown Los Angeles: only about a twenty-minute car ride. On the other hand, to make DHA from ALA is analogous to driving from Los Angeles to Santa Monica by driving to the airport in San Diego and taking a plane to New York, and then another flight back to Seattle. Then from Seattle you would fly to San Francisco, and then take a car to the beach in Santa Monica. You could do it, but it sure would take a lot more time and energy. And that's why until man learned how to scavenge fish (and then eventually fish for them), he wasn't a very smart cookie.

From a molecular point of view, the reason it is so difficult to make DHA from ALA are the requirements of certain enzymes, known as desaturases, represented in the figure above. In particular, to make DHA, ALA has to use the specific enzyme delta-6-desaturase twice. And here lies the problem: ALA tends to decrease the activity of this enzyme. In addition, as you age, the activity of this enzyme decreases. Some DHA eventually gets made from ALA, but it's not an efficient process, as judged by the lower blood levels of DHA in vegetarians. Since the renewal of synaptic junctions (which are rich in DHA) in the brain is constantly taking place, you have to have adequate levels of DHA or the process will be compromised, leading to decreased cognitive skills and less than optimal mental health.

Therefore, if improved cognitive function and mental health are your goals, you are far better off taking oils rich in long-chain Omega-3 fats (fish or algae oils) than you would be by taking oils rich in short-chain Omega-3 fats (like flaxseed oil).

Glossary of Terms

Acerola cherry powder: Acerola, a bush native to the Antilles, is nicknamed the "cherry of the Antilles." When the acerola fruit ripens, it turns red, purple, and yellow; the industry prefers the red fruit. It's lauded for its incredible vitamin C content and is considered a sister to the antioxidant vitamin. The fruit is used in various products such as candies, concentrated juices, preserves, fillings, and medicine tablets and capsules. It can also be purchased in powdered form.

Agar flakes: Agar is a sea vegetable, dried and made into flakes, bars, and powder. It's high in minerals and contains negligible amounts of fat and calories. It's used as an alternative to gelatin, creating the binding necessary in puddings, aspics, tarts, and other desserts. (See **Kanten.**)

Amino acids: The building blocks of proteins. There are 20 amino acids used to construct proteins. The body can't make nine of these amino acids, and therefore they must be supplied by the diet. These are known as essential amino acids. Although amino acids have a slight stimulatory effect on insulin, they have a much more powerful stimulatory effect on glucagon secretion.

Almond butter: See **Nut butters.**

Almond milk: Almond milk is the liquid extracted from ground almonds. Usually, some kind of sweetener is added. Pacific Foods of Oregon is a well-known brand of almond milk.

Amasake or **amazake:** Sometimes flavored with almond or vanilla, amasake is a natural rice-based sweetener with a mild flavor. It's made from sweet brown rice and a bacterial starter called koji—a Japanese cultured food that also is used in making miso, shoyu, and sake, and in pickling. Amasake often comes in "shake" form. It is also used as a sweetener for pies, cakes, puddings, and other desserts.

Anise: An herbaceous plant with a slight licorice flavor.

Apple fiber powder: A fiber or pectin that helps thicken or emulsify ingredients. It is likened to Metamucil because it absorbs toxins in the colon and aids in eliminating waste.

Arrowroot powder: A powder made from the tropical American arrowroot plant. The arrowroot produces a nutritious starch that is used as a thickener in cooking.

Barley: A cereal grain high in Vitamin B, fiber, and protein. After the hull is removed from the grain, the "whole barley" is left, the most nutritious form of the grain. Pearled barley, although more commonly used, has less nutritious value because the second hull is removed in the "pearling" process.

Bok choy: Means "white vegetable" in Cantonese, and is a staple in Chinese cuisine. It has white stalks and broad green leaves. The stalks have a cabbage-like yet sharp taste. The leaves have a milder flavor.

Broccoli rabe (broccoli raab or **rapini):** A kind of broccoli with thin leafy stalks and occasional florets, though this broccoli does not form a "head." It is often used in Italian and Chinese cuisine and appreciated for its aggressive, bitter taste. It's packed with Vitamins A, C, and K and is a good source of potassium.

Button mushrooms: Common, small white mushrooms found in supermarkets.

Canola oil: An oil high in monosaturated fats, made from the rapeseed plant. It has a high burning point and is therefore good for sautéing.

Cardamom: The aromatic seed capsule of a plant native to tropical Asia. It lends a sweet, spicy flavor to foods and is often used in Indian and Asian cuisine.

Chickpeas: Known as garbanzo beans in Spanish, these legumes are small round beans with a tiny pointed tip. They are tan or light yellow, generally, and are often used in salads and soups, or ground to make a thick Middle Eastern spread—hummus.

Cilantro: The Spanish word for fresh coriander. While often the key ingredient in Mexican and southwestern dishes, such as salsas (hence cilantro), it's also called Chinese parsley. (It is popular in Asian cooking.) Its small, green, lacy leaves are cherished for their sprightly, almost citrus-like flavor.

Coriander: Fresh coriander is cilantro (see above). Dried ground coriander maintains a tang of citrus from its fresh form, and a savory quality like sage.

Cumin seed: A small apiaceous plant bearing aromatic, seed-like fruit. The seeds are often ground to a powder. Cumin has a unique, sharp aroma and deep, spicy taste.

Curry: Not actually one spice, but made with upward of 30 different Indian spices, including turmeric, cardamom, ginger, clove, and mace. It is usually bright yellow or mustard-yellow in color.

Daikon: Often called Chinese radish, it comes in two types, white and green, though white is more common. It imparts a radish-like flavor when eaten raw. When cooked, it reveals a natural sweetness. Raw daikon is often shredded to accompany Japanese cuisine, such as sushi.

Dandelion greens: Mostly known as the pesky yellow flowering weeds that pop up after we've mowed the lawn, dandelion greens are very popular in America's South and in Europe. They impart a slightly bitter, yet refreshing taste. They're commonly used in salads, soups, and sauces. They are an excellent source of Vitamin A, and maintain some calcium and iron, and small amounts of potassium and Vitamin C.

Dulse flakes: A seaweed, like kelp, used as a condiment or in cooking. It's also a great source of iron.

Eicosanoids: A very broad group of hormones, derived from essential fatty acids that regulate the internal equilibrium of each cell by sampling the external environment and then interacting with receptors to relay that information back to the cell. Every cell in the body has the ability to make eicosanoids. Excess levels of insulin can induce the body to make more "bad" eicosanoids and fewer "good" ones. The more "bad" eicosanoids that are produced, the more likely you are *to* develop heart disease, cancer, and arthritis.

Essential fatty acids: Fatty acids that the body needs but cannot make, and therefore must be in the diet. They are the building blocks of eicosanoids. There are two groups of essential fatty acids, Omega-6 and Omega-3. Different eicosanoids are produced from these two groups of essential fatty acids.

Fennel: A compact green and white bulb with a distinct licorice flavor. It lends a refreshing sweetness to salads. It's also used in cooking.

Frittata: An Italian term that translates into egg cake made with vegetables.

Fructose powder: Powder made from fructose, which is refined corn syrup.

Garbanzo beans: See **Chickpeas.**

Genistein: The most studied phytoestrogen that is found in soybeans. It can interact with estrogen receptors and inhibit the signaling activity of insulin receptors.

Glucagon: The counterregulatory hormone to insulin that is stimulated by dietary protein. Its primary job is to release stored carbohydrate from the liver to maintain adequate levels of blood sugar for optimal mental performance.

Glycemic index: The rate at which any carbohydrate enters the bloodstream when compared to an equal amount of carbohydrate found in white bread. The lower the glycerine load, the less insulin will be secreted.

Glycemic load: The amount of carbohydrate consumed multiplied by its glycemic index. The total glycemic load of a meal will determine the amount of insulin released after a meal. The lower the glycemic load, the less insulin will be secreted.

High-density carbohydrates: Any carbohydrate that contains a large amount of carbohydrate in a small volume. These more concentrated carbohydrates stimulate rapid insulin secretion. Grains, starches, pasta, and bread products are examples of high-density carbohydrates.

Hummus: A Middle Eastern spread made from chickpeas ground into a paste with olive oil, tahini, lemon, garlic, and sometimes other spices. It makes a great spread or dip and is a good source of protein.

Insulin: The storage hormone secreted by the pancreas in response to carbohydrates, and to a much lesser extent to protein. Fat has no effect on insulin secretion. Insulin's primary job is to drive nutrients into cells for immediate or long-term storage. Excess insulin levels are the primary risk factor for heart disease, Type 2 diabetes, and obesity.

Isoflavones: Phytochemicals that have a cyclic ring structure. Some isoflavones, such as genistein and diadzein, can bind to estrogen receptors and are known as phytoestrogens.

Kanten: A fruit gelatin made by mixing hot water and agar. The mixture is poured over fruit, such as strawberries, cherries, or apricots, and nuts, then refrigerated until firm.

Kelp sea vegetables: Also called kelp. Kelp is a seaweed and, like dulse, is rich in iron. It comes in sheets, dry, and in capsules.

Koji: A live culture of *Aspergillus oryzae* bacteria. It is inoculated into soybeans and sea salt to make miso; it is also used in making amasake, shoyu, sake, and mirin.

Low-density carbohydrates: Any carbohydrate that contains a small amount of carbohydrate in a large volume, such as vegetables.

Macronutrients: Protein, carbohydrate, and fat are macronutrients. Only macronutrients have any effect on hormone secretion. The appropriate balance of protein, carbohydrate, and fat will keep both insulin and glucagon in appropriate zones for a four- to six-hour period.

Mesclun greens: A combination of baby lettuces, such as red oak, arugula, and Lolo Rosa, and bitter lettuces, such as frisee and mild herbs.

Micronutrients: Vitamins and minerals are micronutrients. They act as co-factors used by enzymes in the body and must be supplied by the diet. Without adequate levels of micronutrients, the efficiency of the body's metabolism will decrease.

Mirin: A sweet rice wine used to bring out the flavors in foods.

Miso: A staple of Japanese cuisine for thousands of years. It is a dark paste made of soybeans, unrefined sea salt, and fermented barley or rice. The mixture is cooked, inoculated with koji, a mold that helps aid fermentation, then aged. Miso comes in different types. White, yellow, and tan miso are lighter and sweet. They contain less salt and are aged less. Barley miso, known as *mugi miso*, is made with fermented barley and is mild and mellow. Soybean miso, *hatcho miso,* has a rich, hearty taste. Brown rice miso, *kome miso,* is the sweetest of the misos.

Monounsaturated fats: Fatty acids that do not affect insulin, nor do they adversely affect lipid levels (as do saturated fats). They are the primary fats used in Soy Zone meals.

Mung bean sprouts: Sprouts from the small pea-like mung bean. The sprouts are commonly used in Chinese stir-fry and cuisine.

Nayonaise: Non-dairy mayonnaise made with soy beans and tofu.

Non-aluminum baking powder: Baking powders that contain no sodium aluminum sulphate, often found in double-acting baking powders. Aluminum in the diet is thought to be linked to neurological disorders.

Nut butters: Nut butters, made from ground almonds, hazelnuts, pistachios, or other nuts, and found in health food stores, do not carry the added sugars or preservatives of commercially sold and processed butters, such as peanut butter. One of the sweetest buters is almond butter, which contains a good amount of protein, carbohydrates, and fat.

Nutritional yeast flakes: Like brewer's yeast, nutritional yeast flakes are a great source of Vitamin B. Usually used as a condiment or sprinkled over food, they can be used on popcorn instead of salt. When cooked, yeast flakes lose their nutritional value.

Olive oil: Olive oil is the pressed oil from olives. *Extra-virgin* olive oil is the oil extracted from the first pressing from the olives. Often these olives are superior in quality and the oil maintains a superior quality and flavor. *Virgin* olive oil is made from the second or third pressing of the olives and is often more acidic than extra-virgin. Regular or *pure* olive oil is often processed with solvents and high heat, which often creates an inferior product, both nutritiously and in flavor.

Omega-3 fatty acids: These essential fatty acids include long-chain fatty acids, such as docosahexaenoic acid (DHA), the key to brain function, and eicosapentaenoic acid (EPA), the key to optimal immunological and cardiovascular function. Short-chain Omega-3 fatty acids, such as alpha linolenic acid (ALA), must be metabolized to these longer-chain fatty acids to have a significant impact on the central nervous, immunological, and cardiovascular systems.

Omega-6 fatty acids: The building blocks for both "good" and "bad" eicosanoids. An excess of Omega-6 fatty acids in the diet leads to a buildup of "bad" eicosanoids that accelerate heart disease, Type 2 diabetes, and cancer. High levels of Omega-3 fatty acids inhibit the overproduction of "bad" eicosanoids, derived from Omega-6 fatty acids.

Phytochemicals: Plant compounds that have biological actions.

Phytoestrogens: These are phytochemicals that can interact with the estrogen receptor in cells. In high enough concentrations, phytoestrogens have many of the properties of natural estrogen for women. Soybeans are a rich source of phytoestrogens.

Pistou: A Provençal vegetable soup or stew.

Purified water: Water passed through a purifying or filtering system. Bottled spring water may also be used.

Raita: Traditional Indian dish made with yogurt and cucumbers that cools the palate from spicy foods.

Ramekin: Small soufflé dish usually made out of ceramic or porcelain.

Red barley miso paste: See **Miso**.

Saffron: A brilliant yellow-red herb that imparts color and mild flavor to foods. It comes from the three stigmas and part of the white style of a purple-flowered crocus, which is part of the iris family. Its reputation for being costly is due to the labor-intensive harvest.

Sea salt: Has a higher mineral content than its iodized cousin. It comes coarsely and finely ground.

Shoyu sauce: A brewed soy sauce with a base of soy beans and wheat. It's commonly used in Japan and is considered superior to soy sauce, which is fermented soy beans with salt added.

Soybeans: The only beans that contain more protein than carbohydrate. As a result, food products made from soybeans are richer in protein and therefore ideally suited to balance out carbohydrates for the Soy Zone Diet.

Soy flour: The result of extracting soybeans with hexane to remove the oil. The defatted product is approximately 50 percent protein by weight. Textured vegetable protein (TVP) is made from soy flour.

Soy milk: The liquid from ground soy beans. It is a great source for phytoestrogens, and a good milk substitute for individuals with lactose intolerance.

Soy protein concentrate: The result of extracting soy flour with alcohol to remove much of the carbohydrate, creating a product that is approximately 70 percent protein by weight. Unfortunately, the alcohol extraction also removes the phytoestrogens, which are beneficial for promoting estrogen-like activity and decreasing insulin response.

Soy protein isolate: Water extraction of soy flour produces a soy protein isolate that contains more than 90 percent protein by weight, and retains more of the phytoestrogens, which are beneficial for promoting estrogen-like activity and decreasing insulin response.

Soy Zone Diet: A protein-adequate, carbohydrate-moderate, low-fat diet primarily using soy protein, designed to maintain insulin within a zone (not too high, not too low) from meal to meal.

Stevia extract powder: Stevia is a member of the mint family. It's a sweetener, about 300 times more powerful than sugar. It is used in cooking and baking. Just a drop can sweeten coffee.

Sweet rice wine: See **Mirin.**

Tahini: A mild, sweet sesame paste made from hulled sesame seeds. It's used in sauces, spreads such as hummus, dressings, and custards.

Tamari sauce: This is a shoyu sauce—soy sauce—without the wheat. It has a stronger flavor, but does not undergo the two-year fermentation process that shoyu does.

Tempeh: Pressed fermented soybean cake. It is often steamed, pan-fried, boiled, or broiled. It should never be eaten raw. Its protein content is comparable to that of chicken and beef and contains fiber, the B vitamins, and calcium.

Tofu: Tofu's versatility and high protein content have put it in the celebrity status of American vegetarian meals and other dishes. It is a soybean curd—a "cake" solidified from soybean milk. Chinese tofu consists of bricks of the coagulated curds. Japanese tofu blends the coagulated curds with water-soluble whey protein, creating a custard-like consistency. Chinese tofu tends to be very rich in protein, and is a major component of the Soy Zone Diet. Good-quality tofu will be made with organic soybeans and nigari, a mineral-rich substance. The less water content and the more compressed the cake, the firmer the tofu. The different styles—soft, firm, extra-firm, and smoked—perform different functions in various dishes. Soft tofu is often used for salad dressings and in miso soup and quick-cooking dishes. Firm tofu is often used for heartier applications, such as kebabs, in stir-fry, or deep-fried. Tofu also comes smoked and dried.

Tofu cream: A product made from soybeans.

TVP (textured vegetable protein): A dehydrated soy product often used by vegetarians as a source of protein. It absorbs in bulk water upon heating and is used often in making casseroles and "hamburgers."

Ume paste: Pickled plum paste made from the Japanese umeboshi plum. Often used in macrobiotic diets to aid digestion and stimulates enzyme production.

Umeboshi vinegar: Vinegar made from the juice left over from pickling the tart Japanese umeboshi plums.

Unsweetened juices: Juices extracted from their fruits, such as apple or pineapple, without additives or sweeteners. Sometimes "unsweetened" fruit juices are naturally sweetened from juices of other, sweeter fruits, such as pears or grapes.

Vegetable broth powder: Dehydrated vegetable broth used to make soups and other vegetarian dishes.

Zone Diet: A protein-adequate, carbohydrate-moderate, low-fat diet designed to maintain insulin within a zone from meal to meal.

Zone Food Blocks: An exchange method for macronutrients (protein, carbohydrate, and fat) to prepare meals that maintain the balance of protein and carbohydrate to keep insulin within a defined zone.

Resources

ORGANIZATIONS

American Soybean Association
12125 Woodcrest Executive Drive
Suite 100
Creve Coeur, MO 63141
Tel: 314-576-1770

Soyfoods Association of America
1723 U Street, N.W.
Washington, D.C. 20009
Tel: 202-986-5600

Soyatech
318 Main Street
Bar Harbor, ME 04609
Tel: 207-288-4969

SOYFOOD COMPANIES

Central Soya
1946 W. Cook Road
Fort Wayne, IN 46818
Tel: 219-425-5100
Producers of soy flour, soy protein concentrate, and lecithin.

Eden Foods
701 Tecumseh Road
Clinton, MI 49236
Tel: 517-456-7424
Producers of soy products including soy milk and tofu.

Galaxy Foods
2441 Viscount Row
Orlando, FL 32809
Tel: 407-855-5500
Producers of soy cheese and other dairy analog products, and soy beverages.

Lightlife Foods
74 Fairview Street
Greenfield, MA 01302
Tel: 413-774-6001
Producers of soy meat substitute products, tempeh, and tofu.

Nasoya Foods, Inc.
One New England Way
Ayer, MA 01432
Tel: 978-772-6880
Producers of soy milk products, tofu, and tofu-based products.

NutriSoy International Inc.
424 S. Kentucky Avenue
Evansville, IN 47714
Tel: 888-769-0769
Producers of soy protein concentrate powders.

Protein Technologies
Checkerboard Square
St. Louis, MO 63164
Tel: 314-982-2736
Producers of soy protein isolates.

Vitasoy USA Inc.
400 Oyster Point Blvd.
South San Francisco, CA 94080
Tel: 650-583-9888
Producers of soy milk products and tofu products.

Worthington Foods
900 Proprietors Road
Worthington, OH 43085
Tel: 614-885-9511
Producers of soy meat substitute products.

Yves Veggie Cuisine
1638 Derwent Way
Delta, British Columbia V3M 6R9
Canada
Tel: 604-525-1345
Producers of soy meat substitute products.

LONG-CHAIN OMEGA-3 FATTY ACIDS

Martek Biosciences Corporation
6480 Dobbin Road
Columbia, MD 21045
Tel: 410-740-0081
Producers of algae oils rich in DHA.

Roche Vitamins
45 Waterview Blvd.
Parsippany, NJ 07054
Tel: 800-526-8413
Producers of new high-tech versions of DHA-rich fish oils that are virtually odor-free.

References

Chapter 1: The Health Benefits of Soy

Abertazzi P, Pansini F, Bonaccorsi G, Zamitti L, Forini E, and de Aloysio D "The effect of dietery soy supplement on hot flashes." *Obstet Gynecol* 91: 6–11 (1988).

Akisaka M, Asato L, Chan YC, Suzuki M, Uezata T, and Yamamoto S. "Energy and nutrient intake of Okinawan centenarians." *J Nutr Sci Vitaminol* 42: 241–248 (1996).

———, Suzuki M, and Inoko H. "Molecular genetic studies on DNA polymorphism of the HLA class II genes associated with human longevity." *Tissue Antigens* 50: 489–493 (1997).

American Heart Association. *1997 Heart and Stroke Statistical Update.* Dallas, TX: American Heart Association, 1996.

Anderson JW, Johnstone BM, and Cook-Newell ME. "Meta-analysis of the effects of soy protein intake on serum lipids." *N Engl J Med* 333: 276–82 (1995).

Chatenoud L, La Vecchia C, Francheschi S, Tavani A, Jacobs DR, Parpinel MT, Soler M, and Negri E. "Refined-cereal intake and risk of selected cancers in Italy." *Am J Clin Nutr* 70: 1107–1110 (1999).

Depres J-P, Lamarch B, Mauriege P, Cantin B, Dagenais GR, Moorjani S, and Lupien PJ. "Hyperinsulinemia as an independent risk factor for ischemic heart disease." *N Engl J Med* 334: 952–57 (1996).

Duncan AM, Merz BE, Xu X, Nagel TC, Phipps WR, and Kurzer MS.

"Soy isoflavones exert modest hormonal effects in premenopausal women." *J Clin Endocrinol Metab* 84: 192–97 (1999).

————, Underhill KEW, Xu X, Lavalleur J, Phipps WR, and Kurzer MS. "Modest hormonal effects of soy isoflavones in post-menopausal women." *J Clin Endocrinol and Metab* 84: 3479–84 (1999).

Franceschi S, Favero A, Decarli D, Negri E, La Vecchia C, Ferranroni M, Russo A, Salvini S, Amadori D, Conti E, Montella M, and Giacosa A. "Intake of macronutrients and risk of breast cancer." *Lancet* 347: 1351–1356 (1996).

Ginsburg B and Milken M. *The Taste for Living Cookbook.* Santa Monica, CA: Cap CURE, 1998.

Giovannucci E. "Insulin and colon cancer." *Cancer Causes and Control* 6: 164–179 (1997).

Kagawa Y. "Impact of Westernization on the nutrition of Japanese: Changes in physique, cancer, longevity, and centenarians." *Prev Med* 7: 205–217 (1978).

————, Nishizawa M, Suzuki M, Miyatake T, Hamamoto T, Goto K, Montaonga E, Izumikawa H, Hirata H, and Eibhara A. "Eicospolyenoic acids of serum lipids of Japanese islanders with low incidence of cardiovascular diseases." *J Nutr Sci Vitaminol* 28: 441–453 (1982).

Ludwig DS, Majzoub JA, Al-Zahrani A, Dallal GE, Blanco I, and Roberts SB. "High glycemic index foods, overeating, and obesity." *Pediatrics* 103: E26 (1999).

Markovic TP, Jenkins AB, Campbell LV, Furler SM, Kraegen EW, and Chisholm DJ. "The determinants of glycemic responses to dietetic responses to diet restriction and weight loss in obesity and NIDDM." *Diabetes Care* 21: 687–94 (1994).

McKeown-Eyssen G. "Epidemiology of colorectal cancer revisited: Are serum triglycerides and/or plasma glucose associated with risk?" *Cancer Epidemiology, Biomarkers and Prevention* 3: 687–695 (1994).

Messina V and Messina M. *The Vegetarian Way.* New York: Crown, 1996.

Mimura G, Murakami K, and Gushiken M. "Nutritional factors for longevity in Okinawa—present and future." *Nutr Health* 8: 159–163 (1992).

Mizushima S and Yamori Y. "Nutritional improvement, cardiovascular disease, and longevity in Japan." *Nutr Health* 8: 97–105 (1992).

Mokdad AH, Serdula MK, Dietz WH, Bowman BA, Marks JS, and Koplan JP. "The spread of the obesity epidemic in the United States, 1991–1998." *JAMA* 282: 1519–1522 (1999).

Murkies AL, Lombard C, Strauss BJ, Wilcox G, Burger HG, and Morton MS. "Dietary flour supplementation decreases post-menopausal hot flashes: effect of soy and wheat." *Maturitas* 21: 189–95 (1995).

Okamoto K and Sasaki R. "Geographical epidemiologic studies on factors associated with centenarians in Japan." *Nippon Ronen Igakkai Zasshi* 32: 485–490 (1995).

Potter SM, Baum JA, Teng H, Stillman RJ, and Erdman JW. "Soy protein and isoflavones exert modest hormonal effects on blood lipids and bone density in postmenopausal women." *Am J Clin Nutr* 68: 1375S–1379S (1998).

Sears B. *The Zone.* New York: ReganBooks, 1995.

———. *The Anti-Aging Zone.* New York: ReganBooks, 1999.

Shibata H, Hagai H, Haga H, Yasumura S, Suzki T, and Suyama Y. "Nutrition for the Japanese elderly." *Nutr Health* 8: 165–175 (1992).

Stoll BA. "Essential fatty acids, insulin resistance, and breast cancer risk." *Nutrition and Cancer* 31: 72–77 (1998).

Walford RL. *The 120-Year Diet.* New York: Simon and Schuster, 1986.

——— and Walford L. *The Anti-Aging Plan.* New York: Four Walls Eight Windows, 1994.

Weindruch R and Walford RL. *The Retardation of Aging and Disease by Dietary Restriction.* Springfield, IL: Charles C. Thomas, 1988.

———. "Caloric restriction and aging." *Sci Am* 274: 46–52 (1996).

CHAPTER 2: ENTERING THE SOY ZONE

Adams PB, Lawson S, Sanigorski A, and Sinclair AJ. "Arachidonic acid to eicosapentaenoic acid ratio in blood correlates positively with clinical symptoms of depression." *Lipids* 31: S157–161 (1996).

Agren JJ, Tormala ML, Nenonem MJ, and Haainea OO. "Fatty acid composition of erythrocyte, platelet and serum lipids in strict vegetarians." *Lipids* 30: 365–369 (1995).

Carlson S and Werkman S. "A randomized trial of visual attention of preterm infants fed docosahexanenoic acid until two months." *Lipids* 31: 85–90 (1996).

Connor WE, Neuringer M, and Reisbick S. "Essential fatty acids: The importance of n–3 fatty acids in the retina and brain." *Nutr Rev* 50: 21–29 (1992).

Conquer JA and Holub BJ. "Supplementation with an algae source of docosahexaenoic acid increases (n–3) fatty acid status and alters selected risk factors for heart disease in vegetarian subjects." *J Nutr* 126: 3032–3039 (1996).

Crawford MA, Bloom M, Broadhurst CL, Schmidt WF, Cunnane SC, Galli C, Gehbremeskel K, Linseisen F, Lloyd-Smith J, and Parkington J. "Evidence for the unique function of docosahexaenoic acid during the evolution of the modern hominid brain." *Lipids* 34: S39-S47 (1999).

Hamazaki TS, Sawazaki S, Itomura M, Asaoka E, Nagao Y, Nishimura N, Yazawa K, Kawamori T, and Kobayashi M. "The effect of docosahexaenoic acid on aggression in young adults." *J Clin Investigation* 97: 1129–1133 (1996).

Harris WS. "n–3 fatty acids and serum lipoproteins: human studies." *Am J Clin Nutr* 65: 1645S–1654S (1997).

Hibbeln JR and Salem N. "Dietary polyunsaturated fatty acids and depression: When cholesterol does not satisfy." *Am J Clin Nutr* 62: 1–9 (1995).

Holmes MD, Stampfer MJ, Colditz, Rosner B, Hunter DJ, and Willett WC. "Dietary factors and the survival of women with breast cancer." *Cancer* 86: 751–753 (1999).

Hu FB, Stampfer MJ, Manson JE, Rimm E, Colditz GA, Speizer FE, Hennekens CH, and Willett WC. "Dietary protein and the risk of ischemic heart disease in women." *Am J Clin Nutr* 70: 221–227 (1999).

Kris-Etherton PM, Pearson TA, Wan Y, Hargrove RL, Moriaty K,

Fishell V, and Etherton TD. "High-monounsaturated fatty acid diets lower both plasma cholesterol and triglycerol concentrations." *Am J Clin Nutr* 70: 1009–1015 (1999).

Kyle DJ and Arterburn LM. "Single cell oil sources of docosahexaenoic acid: Clinical studies." *World Rev Nutr Diet* 83: 116–31 (1998).

Lanting CI, Fidler V, Huisman M, Touwen BCL, and Boersma ER. "Neurological differences between 9-year old children fed breast-milk or formula-milk as babies." *Lancet* 344: 1319–1322 (1994).

Lemon P. "Do athletes need more dietary protein and amino acids?" *Int J Sports Nutr* 5: S39–61 (1995).

Makrides M, Neumann M, Simmer K, Pater J, and Gibson RA. "Are long-chain polyunsaturated fatty acids essential nutrients in infancy?" *Lancet* 345: 1463–1468 (1995).

———, Simmer K, Goggin M, and Gibson RA. "Erthyrocyte docosa-hexaenoic acid correlates with the visual response of healthy, term infants." *Pediatric Res* 33:425–427 (1992).

Munger RG, Cerhan JR, and C-H Chiu B. "Prospective study of dietary protein intake and risk of hip fracture in postmenopausal women." *Am J Clin Nutr* 69: 147–152 (1999).

Reddy S, Sanders TB, and Obeid O. "The influence of maternal vegetarian diet on essential fatty acid status of the newborn." *Eur J Clin Nutr* 48: 358–368 (1994).

Rimm EB, Stampfer MJ, Ascherio A, Giovannucci E, Colditz GA, and Willett WC. "Vitamin E consumption and risk of coronary heart disease in men." *N Engl J Med* 328: 1450–1456 (1993).

Sanders TAB and Reddy S. "The influence of a vegetarian diet on the fatty acid composition of milk and the essential fatty acid status of the infant." *J Pediatrics* 120: S71–77 (1992).

Schmidt MA. *Smart Fats.* Berkeley, CA: Frog Ltd., 1997.

Sears B. *The Zone.* New York: ReganBooks, 1995.

———. *Mastering the Zone.* New York: ReganBooks, 1997.

———. *Zone Perfect Meals in Minutes.* New York: ReganBooks, 1998.

———. *Zone Food Blocks.* New York: ReganBooks, 1998.

———. *The Anti-Aging Zone.* New York: ReganBooks, 1999.

Singh A and Ward OP. "Microbial production of docosahexaenoic acid (DHA, C22:6)." *Adv Appl Microbiol* 45: 271–312 (1997).

Skov AR, Toubro S, Ronn B, Holm L, and Astrup A. "Randomized trial on protein vs carbohydrate in ad libitum fat reduced diet for the treatment of obesity." *International Journal of Obesity* 23: 528–536 (1999).

Soderberg M, Edlund C, Kristensson K, and Dallner G. "Fatty acid composition of brain phospholipids in aging and in Alzehimer's disease." *Lipids* 26: 421–425 (1996).

Sprecher H, Chen Q., and Yin F-Q. "Regulation of the biosynthesis of 22:5n–6 and 22:6n–3: A complex intracellular process." *Lipids* 34: S153-S156 (1999).

Stampfer MJ, Hennekens CH, Manson JE, Colditz GA, Rosner B, and Willett WC. "Vitamin E consumption and risk of coronary heart disease in women." *N Engl J Med* 328: 1444–1449 (1993).

Stevens LJ, Zentall SS, and Burgress JR. "Omega–3 fatty acids in boy with behavior, learning, and health problems." *Physiology and Behavior* 59: 915–920 (1996).

———, Zentall SS, Deck JL, Abate ML, Watkins BA, Lipp SR, and Burgress JR. "Essential fatty acid metabolism in boys with attention-deficit hyperactivity disorder." *Am J Clin Nutr* 62: 761–768 (1995).

Stoll AL, Severus E, Freeman MP, Rueter S, Zhoyan HA, Diamond E, Cress KK, and Marangell LB. "Omega–3 fatty acids in bipolar disorder." *Arch Gen Psychiatry* 56: 407–412 (1999).

Swisklocki AM, Chen Y-D, Golay MA, Cheng M-D, and Reaven GM. "Insulin suppression of plasma free fatty acid concentration in normal individuals or patients with type II (non-insulin-dependent) diabetes." *Diabetologia* 30: 622–626 (1987).

Uauy R, Peiremo P, Hoffman D, Mena P, Birch D, and Birch E. "Role of essential fatty acids in the function of the developing nervous system." *Lipids* 31: S167–176 (1996).

Unger RH. "Glucagon and the insulin:glucagon ratio in diabetes and other catabolic illnesses." *Diabetes* 20: 834–838 (1971).

——— and Lefebvre PJ. *Glucagon: Molecular Physiology, Clinical and Therapeutic Implications.* Oxford, England: Pergamon Press, 1972.

Willatts P, Forsyth JS, DiModugno MK, Varma S, and Colvin M. "Effect of long-chain polyunsaturated fatty acids in infant formula on problem solving at 10 months of age." *Lancet* 352: 688–691 (1998).

Young VR. "Protein and amino acid requirements in humans." *Scand J Nutr* 36: 47–56 (1992).

———, Bier DM, and Pellett PL. "A theoretical basis for increasing current estimates of the amino acid requirements in adult man, with experimental support." *Am J Clin Nutr* 50: 80–92 (1989).

CHAPTER 3: ZONING YOUR KITCHEN

Greenberg P. *The Whole Soy Cookbook.* New York: Three Rivers Press, 1998.

Sass L. *Great Vegetarian Cooking Under Pressure.* New York: William Morrow, 1989.

———. *Lorna Sass' Complete Vegetarian Kitchen.* New York: Hearst Books, 1992.

———. *The New Soy Cookbook.* San Francisco: Chronicle Books, 1998.

Sears B. *Zone Perfect Meals in Minutes.* New York: ReganBooks, 1998.

Shurtleff W and Aoyagi A. *The Book of Tofu.* New York: Ballantine, 1975.

CHAPTER 4: SOY ZONE KITCHEN COOKING TIPS

Sass L. *Lorna Sass' Complete Vegetarian Kitchen.* New York: Hearst Books, 1992.

Sears B. *Zone-Perfect Meals in Minutes.* New York: ReganBooks, 1998.

CHAPTER 7: FINE-TUNING THE SOY ZONE DIET

Lemon P. "Do athletes need more dietary protein and amino acids?" *Int J Sports Nutr* 5: S39–61 (1995).

Sears B. *The Zone.* New York: ReganBooks, 1995.

———. *Mastering the Zone.* New York: ReganBooks, 1997.

———. *Zone Food Blocks.* New York: ReganBooks, 1998.

CHAPTER 8: YOUR LONGEVITY REPORT CARD: THE TESTS YOU WANT TO PASS

Scholsberg S and Neporent L. *Fitness for Dummies.* Foster City, CA: IDG Books, 1996.

Sears B. *The Anti-Aging Zone.* New York: ReganBooks, 1999.

CHAPTER 9: INSULIN: YOUR BODY'S DR. JEKYLL AND MR. HYDE

Hollenbeck C and Reaven GM. "Variation of insulin stimulated glucose uptake in healthy individuals with normal glucose tolerance." *J Clin Endocrinol and Metab* 64: 1169–1173 (1987).

Sears B. *The Zone.* New York: ReganBooks, 1995.

———. *The Anti-Aging Zone.* New York: ReganBooks, 1999.

Unger RH. "Glucagon and the insulin:glucagon ratio in diabetes and other catabolic illnesses." *Diabetes* 20: 834–838 (1971).

——— and Lefebvre PJ. *Glucagon: Molecular Physiology, Clinical and Therapeutic Implications.* Oxford, England: Pergamon Press, 1972.

CHAPTER 10: SOY SCIENCE

Adlecreutz H and Mazur W. "Phyto-oestrogens and western diseases." *Ann Med* 29: 95–120 (1997).

Albertazzi P, Pansini F, Bonaccorsi G, Zamitti L, Forini E, and de Aloysio D. "The effect of dietary soy supplementation on hot flashes." *Obstet Gynecol* 91: 6–11 (1998).

Altonn H. "Too much tofu induces brain aging." *Honolulu Star Bulletin,* Nov. 19, 1999.

Anderson JJ and Garner SC. "Phytoestrogens and bone." *Bailliere's Clinical Endocrinology and Metabolism* 12: 543–557 (1998)

Anderson JW, Johnstone BM, and Cook-Newell ME. "Meta-analysis of the effects of soy protein intake on serum lipids." *N Engl J Med* 333: 276–82 (1995).

Anthony MS, Clarkson TB, and Williams JK. "Effects of soy isoflavones on atherosclerosis: potential mechanisms." *Am J Clin Nutr* 68: 1390S–1393S (1998).

Barnes S. "Evolution of the health benefits of soy isoflavones." *Proc Soc Exp Biol Med* 217: 386–392 (1998).

Cassidy A and Griffin B. "Phyto-oestrogens: a potential role in the prevention of CHD?" *Proceedings of Nutr Soc* 58: 193–199 (1999).

Clarkson TB and Anthony MS. "Phytoestrogens and coronary heart disease." *Balliere's Clinical Endocrinology and Metabolism* 12: 589–604 (1998).

Colborn T, Dumanoski D, and Myers JP. *Our Stolen Future.* New York: Dutton, 1996.

Coronary Drug Project Research Group. "The coronary drug project: Findings leading to discontinuation of the 2.5mg/day estrogen group." *JAMA* 214: 1303–1313 (1973).

Duncan AM, Merz BE, Xu X, Nagel TC, Phipps WR, and Kurzer MS. "Soy isoflavones exert modest hormonal effects in premenopausal women." *J Clin Endocrinol Metab* 84: 192–197 (1999).

———, Underhill KEW, Xu X, Lavalleur J, Phipps WR, and Kurzer MS. "Modest hormonal effects of soy isoflavones in postmenopausal women." *J Clin Endocrinol Metab* 84: 3479–3484 (1999).

Divi RL, Chang HC, and Doerge DR. "Anti-thyroid isoflavones from soybean: Isolation, characterization, and mechanisms of action." *Biochem Pharmacol* 15: 1087–1096 (1997).

Forsythe WA. "Soy protein, thyroid regulation and cholesterol metabolism." *J Nutr* 125: 619S–623S (1995).

Gambacciani M, Cappagli B, Piaggesi L, Ciaponi M, and Genazzani AR. "Ipriflavone prevents the loss of bone mass in pharmcological menopause induce by GnRH-agonists." *Calcif Tissue Int* 611: s15-s18 (1997).

Genmari C, Agnusdei D, Crepaldi G, Issaia G, Mazzvoli G, Ortolaandi S, Bufalino L, and Passeri M. "Effect of ipriflavone-a synthetic derivative of natural isoflavones on bone mass loss in the early years after menopause." *Menopause* 5: 9–15 (1998).

Hargreavaes DF, Potten CS, Harding C, Shaw LE, Morton MS, Roberts SA, Howell A, and Bundred NJ. "Two-week dietary soy supplementation has a estrogenic effect on normal premenopausal breast." *J Clin Endocrinol and Metab* 84: 4017–4024 (1999).

Head KA. "Ipriflavone: An important bone-building isoflavone." *Altern Med Rev* 4: 10–22 (1999).

Hodgson JU, Puddely IB, and Beillin LJ. "Supplementation with isoflavoid phytoesterogens does not alter serum lipid concentrations: A randomized trial in humans." *J Nutr* 128: 728–732 (1998).

Jabbar MA, Larrea J, and Shaw RA. "Abnormal thyroid function tests in infants with congenital hypothyroidism: The influence of soy-based formula." *J Am Coll Nutr* 16: 280–282 (1997).

Kapiotis S, Hermann M, Held I, Seelos C, Ehringer H, and Gmeiner BM. "Genistein, the dietary-derived angiogenesis inhibitor, prevents LDL oxidation and protects endothelial cells from damage by atherogenic LDL." *Arterioscler Thromb Vasc Biol* 17: 2868–2874 (1997).

Kim H, Peterson TB, and Barnes S. "Mechanisms of action of the soy isoflavone genistein: Emerging role for its effect via transforming growth factor beta signaling pathways." *Am J Clin Nutr* 68: 1418S–1425S (1998).

Knight DC and Eden JA. "Phytoestrogens-a short review." *Maturitas* 22: 167–175 (1995)

Krimsky S. *Hormonal Chaos.* Baltimore, MD: Johns Hopkins University Press, 2000.

Lakshmanan MR, Neopkroeff CM, Ness GC, Dugan RE, and Porter JW. "Stimulation by insulin of the rat liver beta-hydroxy-beta-methylglutaryl coenzyme A reductase and cholesterol synthesizing activities." *Biochem Biophys Res Comm* 50: 704–710 (1973).

Lichtenstein AH. "Soy protein, isoflavones and cardiovascular disease risk." *J Nutr* 128: 1589–1592 (1998).

Morita T, Oh-hashi A, Takei K, Ikai M, Kasaoka S, and Kiriyama S. "Cholesterol-lowering effects of soybean, potato and rice proteins depend on their low methionine contents in rats fed a cholesterol-free purified diet." *J Nutr* 127: 470–7 (1997).

Moyad MA. "Soy, disease prevention, and prostate cancer." *Semin Urol Oncol* 17: 97–102 (1999).

Murkies AL, Lombard C, Strauss BJ, Wilcox G, Burger HG, and Morton MS. "Dietary flour supplementation decreases post-menopausal hot flashes: Effect of soy and wheat." *Maturitas* 21: 189–195 (1995).

Nepokroeff CM, Lakshmanan MR, Ness GC, Dugan RE, and Porter JW. "Regulation of the dirurnal rhythm of rat liver beta-hydroxy-beta-methylglutaryl coenzyme A reductase activity by insulin, glucagon, cyclic AMP and hydrocortisone." *Arch Biochem Biophys* 160: 387–396 (1974).

Ness GC, Zhao Z, and Wiggins L. "Insulin and glucagon modulate hepatic 3-hydroxy–3-methylglutaryl-coenzyme A reductase activity by affecting immunoreactive protein levels." *J Biol Chem* 269: 29168–29173 (1994).

Nestel PJ, Yamashita T, Sasahara T, Pomeroy S, Dart A, Komesaroff P, Owen A, and Abbey M. "Soy isoflavone improves systemic arterial compliance but not plasma lipids in menopausal and peri-menopausal women." *Arterioscler Thromb Vasc Biol* 17: 3392–3398 (1997).

Potter SM, Baum JA, Teng H, Stillman RJ, and Erdman JW. "Soy protein and isoflavones exert modest hormonal effects on blood lipids and bone density in postmenopausal women." *Am J Clin Nutr* 68: 1375S–1379S (1998).

Sanchez A, Hubbard RW, and Hilton GF. "Hypocholesterolemic amino acids and the insulin glucagon ratio." Sugano M and Beynen AC eds., *Dietary Proteins, Cholesterol Metabolism and Atherosclerosis* (Vol. 16, pp. 126–138). Basel: Krager, 1990.

———, Hubbard RW, and Hilton GF. "Dietary protein control of serum cholesterol by insulin and glucagon." Sugano M and Beynen AC eds., *Dietary Proteins, Cholesterol Metabolism and Atherosclerosis* (Vol. 16, pp. 139–147). Basel: Krager, 1990.

Scheiber MD. "Isoflavones and postmenopausal bone health: A viable alternative to estrogen therapy?" *Menopause* 6: 233–242 (1998).

Sears B. *The Zone.* New York: ReganBooks, 1995.

———. *The Anti-Aging Zone.* New York: ReganBooks, 1999.

Setchell KD, Zimmer-Nechemias L, Cai J, and Heubi JE. "Exposure of infants to phyto-oestrogens from soy-based infant formula." *Lancet* 350: 23–27 (1997).

——— and Cassidy A. "Dietary isoflavones: Biological effects and relevance to human health." *J Nutr* 129: 758S–767S (1999).

Tham DM, Gardner CD, and Haskell WL. "Potential health benefits of dietary phytoestrogens: A review of the clinical, epidemiological, and mechanistic evidence." *J Clin Endocrinol Metab* 83: 2223–2235 (1998).

Unger RH. "Glucagon and the insulin:glucagon ratio in diabetes and other catabolic illnesses." *Diabetes* 20: 834–838 (1971).

——— and Lefebvre PJ. *Glucagon: Molecular Physiology, Clinical and Therapeutic Implications.* Oxford, England: Pergamon Press, 1972.

Washburn S, Burke GL, Morgan T, and Anthony M. "Effect of soy protein supplementation on serum lipoproteins, blood pressure, and menopausal symptoms in perimenopausal women." *Menopause* 6: 7–13 (1999).

Whitten PL, Lewis C, Russell E, and Naftolin F. "Potential adverse effects of phytoestrogens." *J Nutr* 125: 771S–776S (1995).

Williams JK and Clarkson TB. "Dietary soy isoflavones inhibit *in-vivo* constrictor responses of coronary arteries to collagen-induced platelet activation." *Biochem Pharmacol* 54: 759–764 (1998).

CHAPTER 11: HOW THE SOY ZONE DIET STACKS UP AGAINST THE TRADITIONAL VEGETARIAN DIET

Acherio AC, Hennekens CH, and Willett WC. "Trans-fatty acid intake and risk of myocardial infaction." *Circulation* 89: 94–101 (1994).

———, Rimm EB, Giovannucci EL, Spelelman D, Stampfer M, and Willett WC. "Dietary fat and risk of coronary heart disease in men." *Brit Med J* 313: 84–90 (1996).

Alpha Tocopherol, Beta Carotene Cancer Prevention Study Group. "The effect of vitamin E and beta carotene on incidences of lung cancer and other cancers in male smokers." *N Engl J Med* 330: 1029–1035 (1994).

Austin MA, Breslow JL, Hennekens CH, Burning JE, Willett WC, and Krauss RM. "Low-density lipoprotein subclass patterns and risk of myocardinal infarction." *JAMA* 260: 1917–1920 (1988).

Braunwald E. "Cardiovascular medicine at the turn of the millennium: Triumphs, concerns, and applications." *N Engl J Med* 337: 1360–1369 (1997).

Chatenoud L, La Vecchia C, Francheschi S, Tavani A, Jacobs DR, Parpinel MT, Soler M, and Negri E. "Refined-cereal intake and risk of selected cancers in Italy." *Am J Clin Nutr* 70: 1107–10 (1999).

De Lorgeril M, Salen P, Martin J-L, Monaud I, Delaye J, and Mamelle N. "Mediterranean diet, traditional risk factors, and the rate of cardiovascular complications after myocardial infarction: Final report of the Lyon diet heart study." *Circulation* 99: 779–785 (1999).

Depres J-P, Lamarch B. Mauriege P, Cantin B, Dagenais GR, Moorjani S, and Lupien PJ. "Hyperinsulinemia as an independent risk factor for ischemic heart disease." *N Engl J Med* 334: 952–957 (1996).

Fuchs CS, Giovannucci EL, Colditz GA, Hunter DJ, Stampfer MJ, Rosner B, Speizer FE, and Willett WC. "Dietary fiber and the risk of colorectal cancer and adenoma in women." *N Engl J Med* 340: 169–176 (1999).

Gaziano JM, Hennekens CH, O'Donnell CJ, Breslow JL, and Burning JE. "Fasting triglycerides, high-density lipoproteins and risk of myocardial infarction." *Circulation* 96: 2520–2525 (1997).

Ginsburg GS, Sarran C, and Pasternak RC. "Frequency of low serum high-density cholesterol levels in hospitalized patients with 'desireable' total cholesterol levels." *Am J Cardiol* 15: 187–192 (1991).

Giovannucci E. "Insulin and colon cancer." *Cancer Causes and Control* 6: 164–179 (1997).

——— and Willett WC. "Dietary factors and the risk of colon cancer." *Ann Med* 26: 443–452 (1994).

Golay KL, Allaz AF, Morel Y, de Tonnac N, Tankova S, and Reaven G. "Similar weight loss with low-or high-carbohydrate diets." *Am J Clin Nutr* 63: 174–178 (1996).

Gould KL. "Very low-fat diets for coronary heart disease: perhaps, but which one?" *JAMA* 275: 1402–1403 (1996).

———, Ornish D, Scherwitz L, Brown S, Eden RP, Hess MJ, Mullani N, Bolomey L, Dodds F, Armstrong WT, Merritt T, Ports T, Sparler S, and Billings J. "Changes in myocardial perfusion abnormalities by positron emission tomography after long-term, intense risk factor modification." *JAMA* 274: 894–901 (1995).

Harris WS. "n–3 fatty acids and serum lipoproteins: Human studies." *Am J Clin Nutr* 65: 1645S–1654S (1997).

Holmes MD, Hunter DJ, Colditz GA, Stampfer MJ, Hankinson SE, Speizer FE, Rosner B, and Willett WC. "Association of dietary intake of fat and fatty acids with risk of breast cancer." *JAMA* 281: 914–920 (1999).

Hu FB, Stampfer MJ, Manson JE, Rimm E, Colditz GA, Speizer FE, Hennekens CH, and Willett WC. "Dietary protein and risk of ischemic heart disease in women." *Am J Clin Nutr* 70: 221–227 (1999).

Katan MB, Grundy SM, and Willett WC. "Beyond low-fat diets." *N Engl J Med* 337: 563–566 (1997).

Key TJA, Thorogood M, Appleby PN, and Burr ML. "Dietary habits and mortality in 11,000 vegetarians and health conscious people: Results of a 17 year follow up." *Brit Med J* 313: 775–779 (1996).

Krumholtz HM, Seeman TE, Merrill SS, Mendes de Leon CF, Vaccarino V, Silverman DI, Tsukahara R, Ostfield AM, and Berkman LF. "Lack of association between cholesterol and coronary heart disease mortality and morbidity and all-cause mortality in persons older than 70 years." *JAMA* 272: 1335–1340 (1994).

Kushi LH, Folsom AR, Prineas RJ, Misk PJ, Wu Y, and Bostick RM. "Dietary antioxidant vitamins and death from coronary heart disease in post menopausal women." *N Engl J Med* 334: 1156–1162 (1996).

Lamarch B, Tchernof A, Mauriege P, Cantin B, Gagenais GR, Lupien PJ, and Despres J-P. "Fasting insulin and apolipoprotein B levels and low-density particle size as risk factors for ischemic heart disease." *JAMA* 279: 1955–1961 (1998).

Leaf A. "Dietary prevention of coronary heart disease: The Lyon diet heart study." *Circulation* 99: 733–735 (1999).

Ornish D, Scherwitz LW, Billings JH, Gould KL, Merritt TA, Sparler S, Armstrong WT, Ports TA, Kirkeeide RL, Hogeboom C, and Brand RJ. "Intensive lifestyle changes for reversal of coronary heart disease." *JAMA* 280: 2001–2007 (1998).

Rosamond WD, Chambless LE, Folsom AR, Cooper LS, Conwill DE, Clegg L, Wang CH, and Heiss G. "Trends in the incidence of myocardial infarction and in mortality due to coronary heart disease, 1987 to 1994." *N Engl J Med* 339: 861–67 (1998).

Sears B. *The Zone.* New York: ReganBooks, 1995.

———. *The Anti-Aging Zone.* New York: ReganBooks, 1999.

Weindruch R. "Caloric restriction and aging." *Sci Am* 274: 46–52 (1996).

——— and Walford RL. *The Retardation of Aging and Disease by Dietary Restriction.* Springfield, IL: Charles C. Thomas, 1989.

Willett WC, Hunter DJ, Stampfer MJ, Colditz GA, Manson JE, Spiegelman D, Rosner B, Hennekens CH, and Speizer FE. "Dietary fat and fiber in relation to risk of breast cancer." *JAMA* 268 2037–2044 (1992).

CHAPTER 12: FREQUENTLY ASKED QUESTIONS

Abelow BJ, Holford TR, and Inosogna KL. "Cross-cultural association between dietary animal protein and hip fracture: A hypothesis." *Calcif Tissue Inst* 50: 14–18 (1992).

Cassidy CM. "Nutrition and health in agriculturists and hunter-gatherers: A case study of two prehistoric populations." In *Nutritional Anthropology: Contemporary Approaches to Diet and Culture* (pp. 117–146). Bedford Hills, NY: Redgrave, 1980.

Cordain L, Miller J, and Mann N. "Scant evidence of periodic starvation among hunter-gatherers." *Diabetologia* 42: 383–384 (1999).

Cohen MN and Armelagos GJ. "Paleopathology at the origins of agriculture." In Cohen NM and Armelagos GJ eds., *Paleopathology at the Origins of Agriculture*(pp. 585–601). New York: Academic Press, 1984.

Eaton SB and Konner MJ. "Paleolithic nutrition." *N Engl J Med* 312: 283–289 (1985).

———, Shostalle M, and Konner M. *The Paleolithic Prescription.* New York: HarperCollins, 1988.

Folsom AR, Ma J, McGovern PG, and Eckfeldt H. "Relation between plasma phospholipid saturated fatty acids and hyperinsulinemia." *Metabolism,* 45: 223–228 (1996).

Fuchs CS, Giovannucci EL, Colditz GA, Hunter DJ, Stampfer MJ, Rosner B, Speizer FE, and Willett WC. "Dietary fiber and the risk of colorectal cancer and adenoma in women." *N Engl J Med* 340: 169–176 (1999).

Giovannucci E. "Insulin and colon cancer." *Cancer Causes and Control* 6: 164–179 (1997).

———, Rimm EB, Colditz GA, Stampfer MJ, Ascherio A, Chute CC, and Willett WC. "A prospective study of dietary fat and risk of prostate cancer." *J Natl Cancer Inst* 85: 1571–1579 (1993).

Holmes MD, Stampfer MJ, Colditz GA, Rosner B, Hunter DJ, and Willett WC. "Dietary factors and the survival of women with breast cancer." *Cancer* 86: 751–753 (1999).

Jain SK, Kannan K, and Lim G. "Ketosis (acetoacetate) can generate oxygen radicals and cause increased lipid peroxidation and growth inhibition in human endothelial cells." *Free Radical Biol and Med* 25: 1083–1088 (1998).

——— and McVie R. "Hyperketonemia can increase lipid peroxidation and lower glutathione levels in human erthrocytes in vitro and in Type 1 diabetic patients." *Diabetes* 48: 1850–1855 (1999).

———, McVie R, Jackson, R, Levine SN, and Lim G. "Effect of hyperketonemia on plasma lipid peroxidation levels in diabetic patients." *Diabetes Care* 22: 1171–1175 (1999).

Kern PA, Ong JM, Soffan B, and Carty J. "The effects of weight loss on the activity and expression of adipose-tissue lipoprotein lipase in very obese individuals." *N Engl J Med* 322: 1053–1059 (1990).

Key TJA, Thorogood M, Appleby PN, and Burr ML. "Dietary habits and mortality in 11,000 vegetarians and health conscious people: Results of a 17 year follow up." *Brit Med J* 313: 775–779 (1996).

Kritchevsky D. "Protein requirements of the elderly." In Munro H and Schlierf A, eds., *Nutrition of the Elderly* (Nestle Nutrition Workshop Series Vol. 20; pp. 81–90). New York: Raven Press, 1992.

McKeown-Eyssen G. "Epidemiology of colorectal cancer revisted: Are serum triglycerides and/or plasma glucose associated with risk?" *Cancer Epidemiology, Biomarkers and Prevention* 3: 687–695 (1994).

Messina V and Messina M. *The Vegetarian Way.* New York: Crown, 1996.

Moore FM. *Diet for a Small Planet.* New York: Ballantine, 1971.

Munger RG, Cerhan JR, and C-H Chiu B. "Prospective study of dietary protein intake and risk of hip fracture in postmenopausal women." *Am J Clin Nutr* 69: 147–152 (1999).

Schuette SA, Zemel MB, and Linkswiler HM. "Studies on the mechanisms of protein-induced hypercalciuria in older men and women." *J Nutr* 110: 305–315 (1980).

Sears B. *The Anti-Aging Zone.* New York: ReganBooks, 1999.

Storlien LH, Jenkins AB, Chisholm DJ, Pascoe WS, Khouri S, and Kraegen EW. "Influence of dietary fat composition on development of insulin resistance in rats. Relationship to muscle triglyceride and omega–3 fatty acids in muscle phospholipid." *Diabetes* 40: 280–289 (1991).

———, Pan DA, Kriketos AD, O'Connor J, Caterson ID, Cooney GJ, Jenkins AB, and Baur LA. "Skeletal muscle membrane lipids and insulin resistance." *Lipids* 31: S261–265 (1996).

Weindruch R. "Caloric restriction and aging." *Sci Am* 274: 46–52 (1996).

——— and Walford RL. *The Retardation of Aging and Disease by Dietary Restriction.* Springfield, IL: Charles C. Thomas, 1988.

Young VR. "Protein and amino acid requirements in humans." *Scand J Nutr* 36: 47–56 (1992).

———, Bier DM, and Pellett PL. "A theoretical basis for increasing current estimates of the amino acid requirements in adult man, with experimental support." *Am J Clin Nutr* 50: 80–92 (1989).

CHAPTER 13: WORLD HEALTH IMPLICATIONS FOR THE SOY ZONE DIET

Eaton SB and Konner MJ. "Paleolithic nutrition." *N Engl J Med* 312: 283–289 (1985).

———, Shostalle M, and Konner M. *The Paleolithic Prescription.* New York: HarperCollins, 1988.

Moore FM. *Diet for a Small Planet.* New York: Ballantine, 1971.

Rifkin J. *Beyond Beef.* New York: Dutton, 1993.

Robbins J. *Diet for New America.* Walpole, NH: Stillpoint, 1987.

APPENDIX B: ZONE VALIDATION STUDIES

Ludwig DS, Majzoub JA, Al-Zahrani A, Dallal GE, Blanco I, and Roberts SB. "High glycemic index foods, overeating, and obesity." *Pediatrics* 103: E26 (1999).

Markovic TP, Jenkins AB, Campbell LV, Furler SM, Kraegen EW, and Chisholm DJ. "The determinants of glycemic responses to diet restriction and weight loss in obesity and NIDDM." *Diabetes Care* 21: 687–94 (1998).

Sears B, Kahl P, and Rapier G. "A nutrition intervention program to improve glycemia, lipid profiles, and hyperinsulinemia in patients with type 2 diabetes." *Diabetes Care* 21: A21 (1998).

APPENDIX D: ZONE FOOD BLOCKS FOR MAKING SOY ZONE MEALS

Foster-Powell K and Miller JB. "International tables of glycemic index." *Am J Clin Nutr* 62: 871S–893S (1995).

Jenkins DJA, Wolever TMS, Taylor RH, Barker H, Fielden H, Baldwin JM, Bowling AC, Newman HC, Jenkins AL, and Goff DV. "Glycemic index of foods: physiological basis for carbohydrate exchange." *Am J Clin Nutr* 34: 362–366 (1981).

Wolever TMS, Jenkins DJA, Jenkins AL, and Josse RG. "The glycemic index: Methodology and clinical implications." *Am J Clin Nutr* 54: 846–854 (1991).

APPENDIX F: GLOSSARY OF TERMS

Kilham, CS. *The Bread & Circus Whole Food Bible.* Addison-Wesley, 1991.

Kimball C. *The Cook's Bible.* Little, Brown, 1996.

Kushi M. *Macrobiotic Diet.* Japan Publications, 1993.

Lo San R. *Bok Choy and Beyond.* Artisan, 1996.

Schneider E. *Uncommon Fruits & Vegetables: A Common Guide.* Harper & Row, 1986.

Seddon G, and Burrow J. *The Natural Food Book.* Rand McNally, 1977, 1980.

Webster's New Universal Unabridged Dictionary. Dilithium Press, 1989.

index

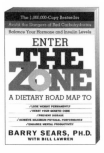
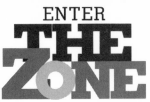
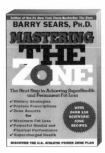
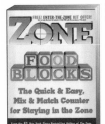
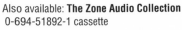